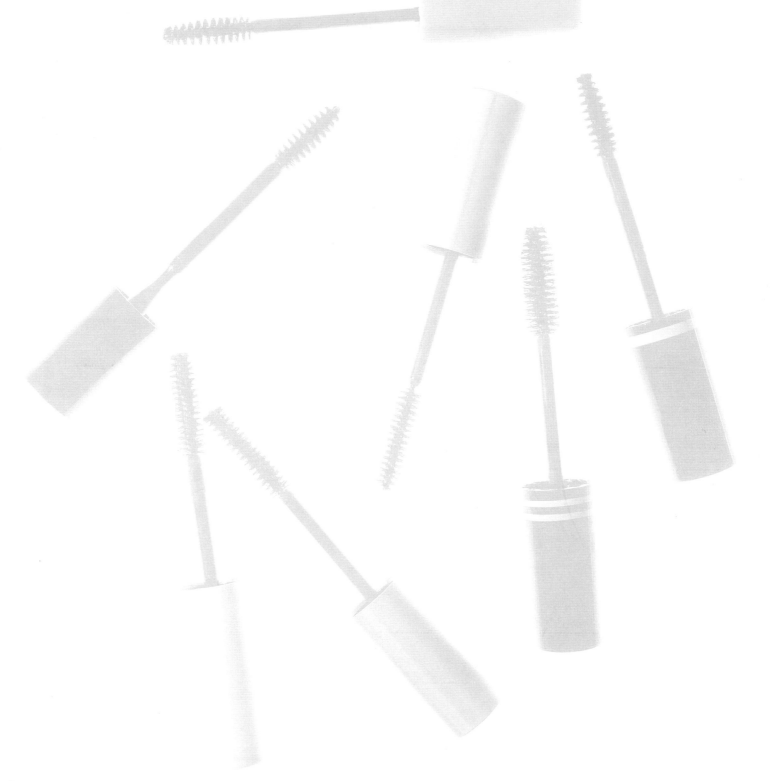

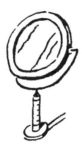

"Show me a woman who is prouder of her clean kitchen than of her collection of lingerie and I'll show you a woman with enlarged pores."

CYNTHIA HEIMEL, *Sex Tips for Girls*

CHIC
SIMPLE ®

WOMAN'S FACE

SKIN CARE *and* MAKEUP

ALFRED A. KNOPF   NEW YORK   1997

THIS IS A BORZOI BOOK
PUBLISHED BY ALFRED A. KNOPF, INC.

Grateful acknowledgement is made to Warner Bros. Publications U.S. Inc. for permission to reprint an excerpt from "Don't It Make My Brown Eyes Blue" by Richard Leigh,
copyright © 1976, 1977 by EMI U Catalog Inc. All rights reserved. Reprinted by permission of Warner Bros. Publications U.S. Inc., Miami, FL 33014.

KIM JOHNSON GROSS   JEFF STONE
WRITTEN BY RACHEL URQUHART
MAKEUP AND EDITORIAL CONSULTING BY LIZ MICHAEL
DESIGN BY DREW SOUZA

PHOTOGRAPHS BY GENTL & HYERS
STYLING BY JULIA BAIER
ILLUSTRATIONS BY LAURIE ROSENWALD
ICON ILLUSTRATIONS BY AMY JESSICA NEEDLE
MIRROR ICON ILLUSTRATION BY ERIC HANSON
PHOTOGRAPHY CONSULTING BY WAYNE WOLF

Library of Congress Cataloging-in-Publication Data
Gross, Kim Johnson.
Woman's face/[Kim Johnson Gross, Jeff Stone, Rachel Urquhart].
p. cm.—(Simple chic)
ISBN 0-679-44578-1 (hc)
1. Beauty, Personal. 2. Face—Care and hygiene. I. Stone, Jeff, II. Urquhart, Rachel. III. Title. IV. Series.
RA778.G8657 1997
646 7'2—dc21
97-5164
CIP

Printed and bound in Great Britain by
Butler & Tanner Ltd, Frome and London
First Edition

A special thanks to Liz Michael, who so patiently shared her makeup wisdom with us, and to Shelley, who FACES us daily and still looks radiant.

K.J.G. & J.S.

For Glenna and Carolyn, natural beauties who have always enjoyed the fun of making up.

K.J.G.

For Ruth and Nan, timeless beauties. Even Helen of Troy was jealous, not that either of you knew her personally.

J.S.

For Theo, my favorite face.

R.U.

The most valuable beauty tip I can give anyone is to accept your face.

L.M.

"The more you know, the less you need."

AUSTRALIAN ABORIGINAL SAYING

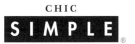

CHIC
SIMPLE

Chic Simple is a primer for living well but sensibly. It's for those who believe that quality of life comes not in accumulating things but in paring down to the essentials. Chic Simple enables readers to bring value and style into their lives with economy and simplicity.

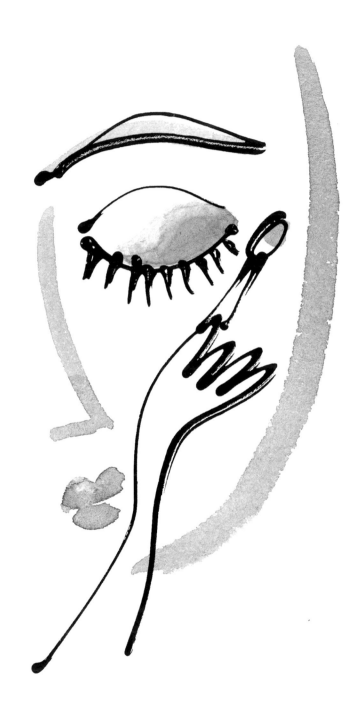

CONTENTS

HOW TO USE THIS BOOK: With each look into the mirror, there are a thousand variables that face you. What you need is a method of understanding and discerning what's important to you. We try to help you ask the questions and, even more important, find the answers. To guide you quickly, we've developed the following icons as mileposts to key information throughout our books. They either highlight answers or refer to the place in the book where you can find additional information.

I C O N S

BASIC. Survival gear, must-haves, or just the BASIC makeup building blocks, these are the essential items that will allow you instant confidence.

COLOR. This icon calls attention to a COLOR issue—both for your individual palette and when it's used to add sizzle.

FAQ. Who? What? Why? When? Here are the answers to the most FREQUENTLY ASKED QUESTIONS (acronym courtesy of the Net).

FIRST AID. To use a euphemism, "something" always happens, so follow the page number to the back of the book for preventive medicine and remedies for makeup misfortunes.

HOW TO. Everyone needs a little help with something—even RuPaul. Whether it's putting on fake eyelashes or finding the perfect moisturizer, here's how to do it with authority.

ON THE ROAD. Travel is a way of life today, and simplifying your beauty routine can ease the long, strange trip it can be.

PERSONAL STYLE. Step-by-step guides to help you try on new looks—and to help you land on that ideal personal style.

PROFILE. Throughout the long journey of style there have been certain individuals, companies, and even products that stand out as important design milestones.

SIMPLE TRUTHS. Wisdom and pieces of advice to help make life simpler. It's a fact: earrings shouldn't weigh more than your head, eyelashes shouldn't enter a room before you do, plus other clarifications.

SKIN. Your skin type will determine whether a product will work for you or not. Look to the lizard. It never lies (except in the sun).

TEXTURE. COLOR and TEXTURE are the key elements that add to your visual impact. Different textures, especially when expertly playing against each other, bring added dimension, not to mention extra versatility, to your look.

VALUE. Invest in VALUE. Which doesn't always mean buying what costs the least. Find out where you should invest and where you can skimp.

Everything you need to know to simply look your best

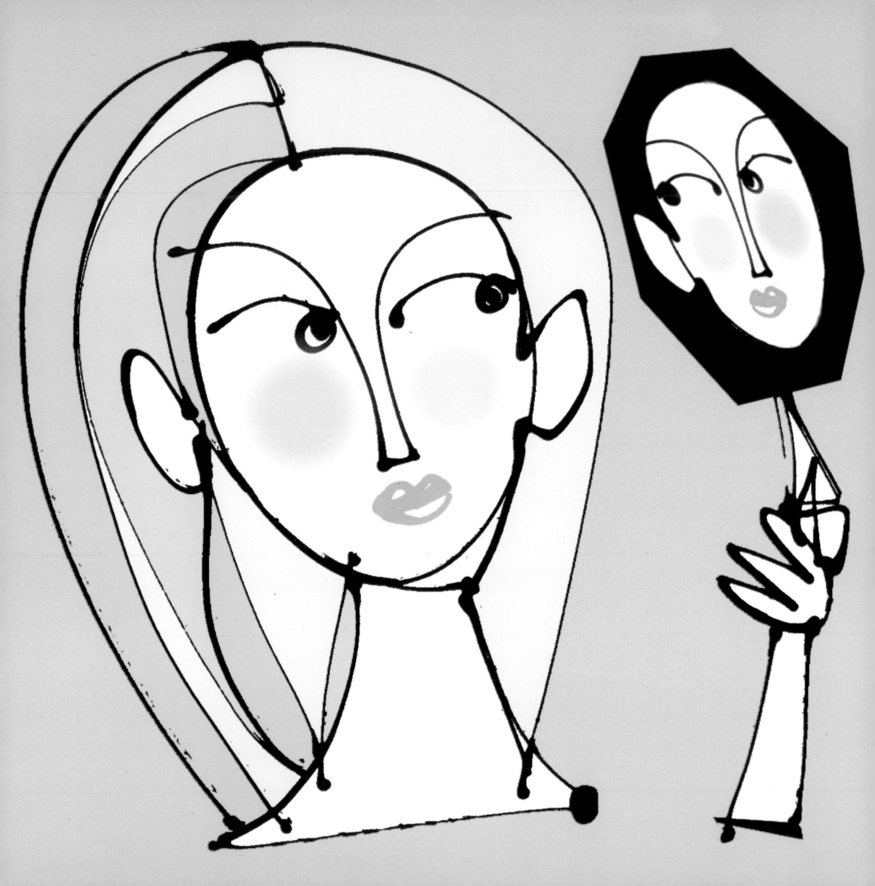

Looking Good

"YES, SHE WAS PRETTY, DISTINCTLY PRETTY; AND TO-NIGHT HER FACE SEEMED REALLY VIVACIOUS. SHE HAD THAT LOOK THAT NO WOMAN, HOWEVER HISTRIONICALLY PROFI-CIENT, CAN SUCCESSFULLY COUNTERFEIT—SHE LOOKED AS IF SHE WERE HAVING A GOOD TIME."

F. SCOTT FITZGERALD, *"Bernice Bobs Her Hair"*

UNDERSTANDING YOUR NEEDS

As the old song goes, looking good is about accentuating the positive and eliminating the negative. It demands that we take stock. What do we like and dislike about our appearance? How do we live? Do we have the time and budget for elaborate skin-care routines, or do our patience and pocketbook extend only to the most basic splash-and-dry regimen? How, exactly, do we feel about makeup anyway? This book walks you through the basics. It helps you audit your life to determine what you want, what you need, and what your time and budget will allow. It addresses complexion type, skin care, and the fundamentals of makeup. It also shows you the specifics, from how to apply eyeshadow to what colors and textures work best for your skin. Looking your best requires some research and experimentation. What follows is a guide to help you get the job done and have some fun along the way.

"If I had to get by on nothing but a pretty face,
I'd drown myself."

ANNA MAGNANI

Feel good in your skin?

WHEN WE LOOK GOOD, WE FEEL GOOD. OR SO THEY TELL US. IT'S ABOUT GOOD HEALTH, IT'S ABOUT CONFIDENCE, IT'S ABOUT ENJOYING THE JOURNEY WE ARE ON. WE STAND TALLER, PROJECT OUR VOICES BETTER. We feel, as the French say, "good in our skin." It's about feeding mind and body with the nourishment they need to light us from within. We need to treat our skin with the respect it deserves, coddling it through harsh weather, accepting the effects of aging, and, of course, forgiving the occasional indulgence in one excess or another. We may choose to dress our face in makeup just as we wrap our body in fine fabrics, or soothe and nourish it with seaweed and herbs. And the end result? Poise. Composure. Feeling good about facing the world. And why not?

HOW TO **CONFIDENCE.** It can have many immediate returns, among them a decrease in stress, a better chance of landing a job, even a lowered statistical likelihood of getting mugged. And as you see how much better it makes you feel, you gain one more thing still: more confidence. **POSTURE.** If you were a jellyfish, maybe you'd have an excuse for slinking about. But you have a spine, so show it off. Standing upright is one of the most important signals that you're sure of yourself. **HANDSHAKE.** Are you shaking someone's hand or slipping them a wet noodle? A firm handshake (try not to crush any bones) and good eye contact say you're relaxed. **EYE CONTACT.** Looking people straight in the eye when you're speaking to them is the ideal way to get your point across: you believe in what you're saying. Good eye contact can also make you a better listener. **VOICE.** Your tone of voice betrays how you're feeling even before you finish your sentence. Like the handshake, a voice of confidence is warm but firm; it avoids the clamminess of whining and the hand buzzer of hysteria. **SMILE.** Yes, fashion models pout. But that's because they're hungry. Yes, smiling may cause wrinkles, but so will frowning. An easy smile is a much-overlooked asset in today's intense world. It means you're confident enough not to always have to take things so seriously. **LAUGH.** Laughing is (almost) the ultimate release. It comes from deep within you. If you have an easy laugh, you show beyond a shadow of a doubt that you can enjoy yourself and others. You'll also reduce stress in the process. **GROOMING.** Taking care of your skin, your teeth, and your hair is a matter of self-respect on the most basic level. The rest is window dressing.

nurture

THE FIRST STEP IS TAKING STOCK OF YOUR SKIN. WHO ARE YOU? WHAT ARE YOUR SKIN'S ASSETS AND liabilities? What makes your skin unique? What are the specifics of your life—diet, exercise, job, habits both naughty and nice—that affect your skin? And consider the factors you can't change: the complexion you were born with, your skin's sensitivity to the sun, the proximity of your capillaries to the top layer of your skin. What is your current skin-care regimen? Does it feel good? Do you like the results? How much time and money are you willing to spend on finding a better one? After you've done an initial audit of your skin, the second step is getting serious about maintenance.

HOW TO **CLEANING.** First you have to remove your makeup—another skin-specific process. Then wash your face gently but thoroughly with tepid water and a cleanser that fits your skin type. You'll need to cleanse at least once a day, right before bedtime, and you may also need a second light washing in the morning. But remember that overcleansing can strip your skin of its natural emollients and lead to increased oil production. The next step is **MOISTURIZING.** Moisturizers do not actually add moisture to your skin, but for most people they are helpful in preventing dryness and irritation, and maintaining skin that is smooth, soft, and supple. And finally, **PROTECTING** your face from this harsh world. It needs a break from sun, cold, excess dryness, and polluted air. Creams and lotions with SPFs (sun-protection factors) and vitamins can help.

FALSE ASSUMPTIONS. Chances are, the skin type you think you have is the result of what you put on it. You may assume you have dry skin, not realizing that your cleanser is stripping away your skin's natural oil. You may think you have oily skin because it's breaking out, when the real culprit is your moisturizer. To find out what kind of skin you really have, use the bare minimum of skin-care products for a few weeks. Wash with warm water and a mild cleanser. Don't moisturize unless you have to. This is also helpful for sensitive skin that's been overloaded with products that are irritating. Get your skin working on its own, so that you can evaluate where it might need a little extra help.

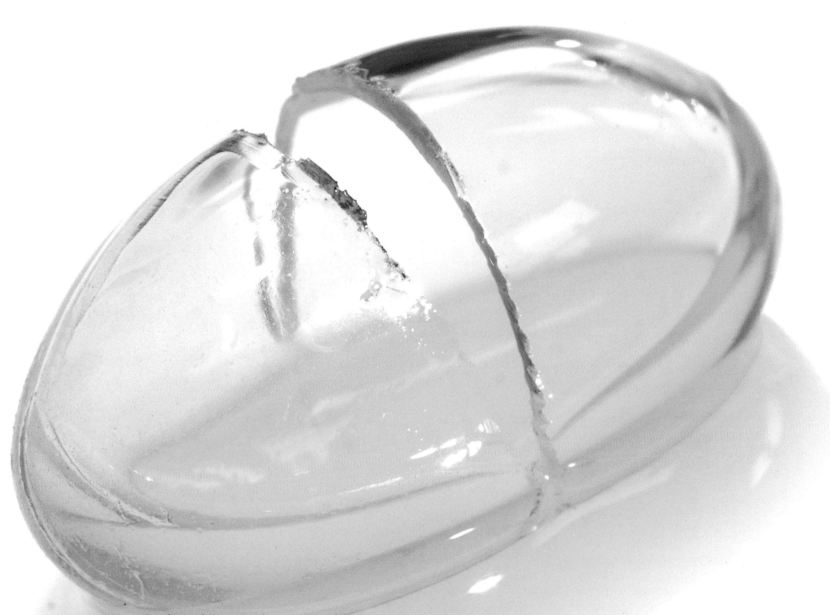

VITAMIN E. The first of the wonder vitamins for skin, vitamin E has range. When applied directly to the skin (but never to broken skin or open cuts), it can lighten scars and help soften and heal chapped lips and ragged cuticles. It can be dabbed over lipstick to give a glossy finish. Taken as a vitamin supplement, E can increase the body's natural sun-protection factor and strengthen the structure of the skin by helping to fight corrosive free radicals.

[🔖 VITAMINS *first aid—page 169*]

Almost everyone hates something about their face. Their nose is too big or too small. Their cheeks are too full or too hollow. And their mouth? So thin, so fat, so long, so pursed— you fill in the blank. **YET "FLAWS" OFTEN BECOME THE VERY THINGS THAT MAKE US BEAUTIFUL.** Look at Lauren Hutton's gap teeth, Cindy Crawford's mole, Anjelica Huston's prominent nose. Enhance your best features, and remember that what you perceive to be minuses may well be pluses.

WHY BOTHER?

BECAUSE. BECAUSE IT MAKES US FEEL PRETTY, LIKE PUTTING ON A PARTY DRESS. BECAUSE IT MAKES US FEEL STRONG, LIKE SLIPPING INTO A COAT OF ARMOR AS THIN AND comfortable as a second skin. Because it gives us the control to celebrate our pros and camouflage our cons. Call it confidence in a compact, flair in a tube. Makeup gives us the sense that we are putting forward not only our best foot, but our best face. Keeping our skin in great shape is just the beginning. The exact shade, texture, and amount of makeup we apply after that depend on lots of things. It can get personal, taking into account our age, coloring, and skin type. And there's mood and personal style to be considered. What's the weather like? Where are we—on safari in Africa or in a café on Place des Victoires? What exactly are we getting ourselves all dolled up for—a holiday gathering or a touch football game? Finally, how do we feel at any one particular moment? We may simply want to luxuriate in the routine of washing and caring for our skin. Or, with brushes and Q-Tips at the ready, we may look at our naked faces as the ultimate creative challenge.

what do you do?

UNFORTUNATELY, IT'S NOT ALWAYS POSSIBLE TO PUT YOUR BEST FACE FORWARD EVERY DAY. MAYBE YOU SLEPT WITH YOUR HEAD JAMMED BETWEEN THE MATTRESS AND THE WALL. MAYBE YOU DIDN'T SLEEP A WINK.

Maybe you had one too many margaritas last night. Whatever the cause, somebody replaced the mirror in the bathroom with a Braque print, and it's not funny at all. On these days the dilemma you face may be dark under-eye circles, a breakout, or an eerie overall sallowness. Take it as an IOU from the grand wheel of facial karma for a good day in the future, but for now the matter at hand is damage control. Try taking a brisk walk around the block to give you a little color and make you feel better all over. A nap can also work wonders, or a nice soak in the tub with a warm washcloth or cotton pads dipped in witch hazel over your eyes. Then there are the cosmetic approaches: consider a quick exfoliation or a nourishing facial mask. Concealer can be a friend here, but don't wear more makeup than you normally do: your ruse will be detected. Instead, you might try a little bronzer to lend your face a warm glow. Also, drink a lot of water. You'll look fine tomorrow.

"I never forget a face, but in your case I'll make an exception."

GROUCHO MARX

• ▮▮ your laundry. • Take a bubble bath. • Rent ▮

movie. • Call in sick. • Wear all black and hole up

in a coffee shop. • Go to the gym. • Avoid brightly

lit areas. • Work from home. • Hide everybody's

eyeglasses. • Make a lot of phone calls. • Start writing

your novel. • Drink some herbal tea—ginger root or mint

BAD FACE DAY

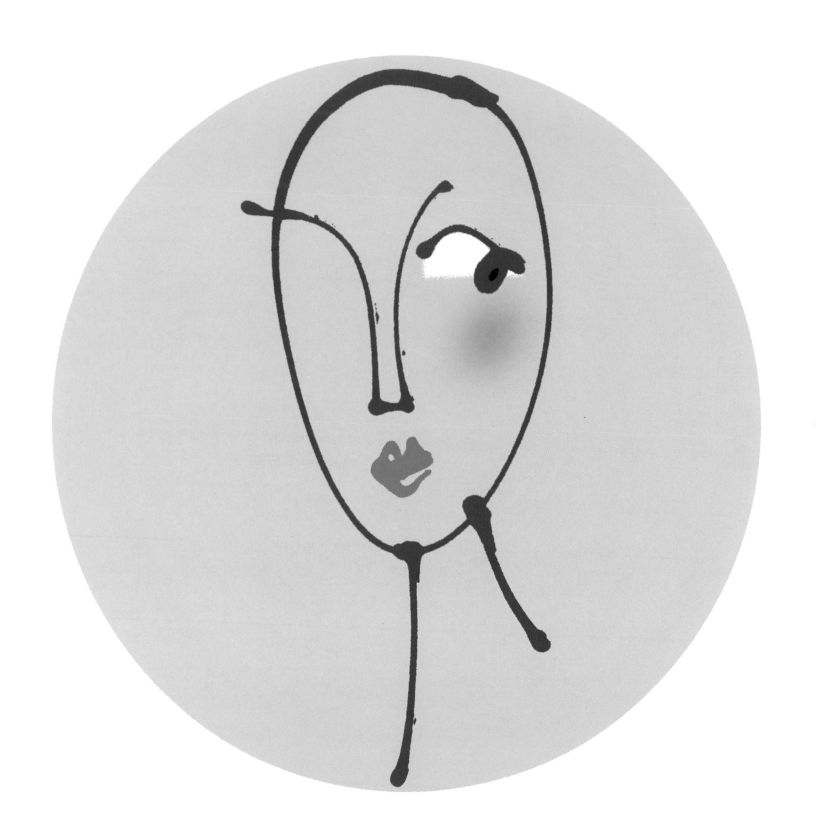

CHAPTER 2

Understanding Your Skin

What can I do to keep my skin healthy? [page 29]   How does my life-style affect my skin? [page 29]   How can I determine what my skin type is? [page 33]   What's the best, easiest way to take care of my skin? [page 34]   Do my skin's needs change as I get older? [page 42]

"A girl came in the café and sat by herself at a table near the window. **She was very pretty, with a face fresh as a newly minted coin,** if they minted coins in smooth flesh with rain-freshened skin."

ERNEST HEMINGWAY, *A Moveable Feast*

F A C I N G   F A C T S

It is your body's largest organ, a thin, resilient barrier between you and the outside world. It protects you from UV rays, pollution, and smoke. It excretes wastes, regulates your body temperature, and distributes nutrients and oxygen to your nerves, glands, hair, and nails. It affords you a sense of touch. Still, we take it for granted—especially the vulnerable skin on our face. It needs care. Start on the inside, with proper diet and exercise. Steer clear of the sun, cigarettes, and stress. Decode the combination of genetics and shifting environment that makes your skin exclusively yours, and treat it accordingly. It may mean an adjustment in your current skin-care regimen, but it's worth it. After all, you've got only one face.

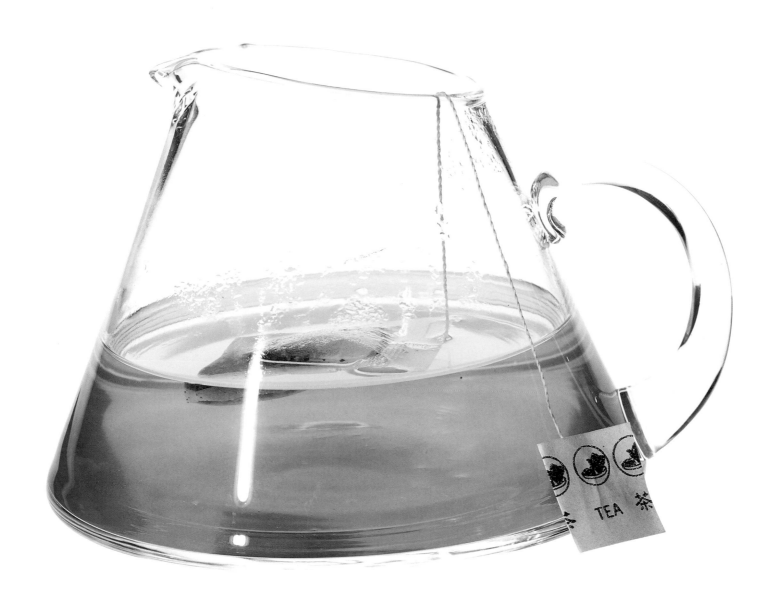

SLEEPING BEAUTY. Like the other major organs of the body, the skin repairs itself while you're sleeping. A normal sleep cycle enables your body to maintain a normal hormonal cycle, which is inextricably tied to healthy skin. On top of that, when you are rested, you are less likely to experience stress, which also can have a negative effect on skin. You'll also have less of a chance of bumping into a wall, which doesn't do wonders for the face, either. And don't overlook other simple remedies: **GREEN TEA** is a stimulant and wrinkle-fighting antioxidant. **CHAMOMILE TEA** is soothing, and you can place the tepid tea bags on your eyelids to reduce puffiness.

[🌿 SKIN TALK *first aid—page 168*]

Inside

THERE ARE THE PROBLEMS WE ARE BORN WITH...AND THEN THERE ARE THOSE WE CREATE FOR ourselves. When it comes to determining things like sun sensitivity, skin type, and susceptibility to wrinkles, our genes hold the cards. But DNA doesn't account for everything. There's a school of thought that says that how we live and feel about ourselves has a greater impact on our complexion than does our genetic blueprint. Diet, exercise, and stress all play important roles. Don't be passive. Education is the key. You have the power to change any number of habits—from that annoying addiction to cheese puffs to the way you clean your face—that will affect the look of your skin.

HORMONES. Estrogen keeps the skin metabolically active, soft, and well hydrated. At high levels—when you are on the Pill, for example—it can also lead to uneven pigmentation of the skin. As levels drop off—during and after menopause—cell renewal slows down, and skin can become dry and more vulnerable to environmental damage. The relatively higher level of testosterone can cause larger pores, increased oil production, and more facial hair. Gentle exfoliating, cleansing, and moisturizing are particularly important now. **STRESS.** It may not take much to send your adrenal glands into overdrive, releasing hormones that stimulate oil production in the sebaceous glands. Get some exercise. It will help you blow off steam, increase the blood flow to your face, and expel toxins through your pores. **ALCOHOL.** A glass of wine or two hasn't been found to be bad for your skin, although red wine is thought to be worse than other alcoholic beverages if you have very sensitive skin with broken veins or rosacca. Heavy drinking is another story: it causes the constant dilation of tiny veins in the face, which can lead to a permanent network of purplish-red capillaries, especially across the nose and cheeks. **DIET.** A body starved of nutrients disintegrates alarmingly quickly. Crazy diets can lead to dehydration and malnutrition, which show up in the skin and as hair and nail loss, an increased number of infections, and bleeding gums. If you need to lose weight, restrict calories, not nutrients. Try to drink eight 8-ounce glasses of noncaffeinated liquid a day (caffeine and alcohol cause dehydration by putting your kidneys into overdrive). **EXERCISE.** Exercise increases circulation and aids in the distribution of nutrients and oxygen to the skin. Sweating also helps free grime from your skin. At the very least, you'll have a healthy glow.

Outside

WHEN YOU THINK ABOUT IT, WE SHOULD BE PLATED LIKE ARMADILLOS. CARS AND SMOKESTACKS BELCH PORE-CLOGGING FILTH. THE SUN SHRIVELS AND BURNS US. THE COLD CHAPS AND PARCHES US. OUR SKIN TELLS

the tale. At times, there seems to be nowhere to hide. Or is there? **POLLUTION AND SMOKING.** The war is on free radicals, the highly reactive chemicals that scramble the molecular makeup of our skin, causing a kind of dermal rusting. Next to sunlight, smoking is the primary culprit, although an adrenaline rush can also generate the rogue electrons. They starve skin tissues of oxygen, causing premature aging. Pollution further asphyxiates the skin by attaching to

What are the effects of smoking on the skin? Smoking is the second major cause of wrinkles, after sun exposure. Nicotine constricts the skin's small blood vessels and decreases the flow of oxygen and nutrients to the epidermis. Some, but certainly not all, smoking-caused wrinkles occur around the mouth from repeatedly pursing the lips around a cigarette. Smoking also slows wound recovery and stains the skin.

hemoglobin in the blood and preventing oxygen flow. Vitamins E, C, and A and beta-carotene are antioxidants and help to combat environmental damage. They can be taken internally as supplements, and are also found in certain moisturizers. **CLIMATE CONTROL.** We take shelter from zero-degree blizzards in stifling office towers. We fend off the stultifying heat of the tropics with blasts of dry, icy air conditioning. Our skin copes with extremes of climate, but pays the price.

smoking, drinking, sunbathing, staying up late, lying to your mother, bacon, guilt, cussing, cheating at Scrabble, sugar

What Kind of Skin Do You Have?

FOR BETTER OR WORSE, WE ALL HAVE DIFFERENT KINDS OF SKIN AND, THEREFORE, DIFFERENT NEEDS: NORMAL, OILY, DRY, SENSITIVE, OLDER, OR A COMBINATION OF THESE. WHAT'S YOUR SKIN TYPE? YOU BE THE JUDGE.

Normal • Your skin burns first, then tans • Your skin tone is fair to medium • Your skin breaks out occasionally, especially in the T-zone • Your pores are larger in the T-zone • Your cheeks feel slightly tight just after cleansing • Your cheeks get dry and chapped • As you get older, you will have a few lines around your eyes, forehead, and upper lip **Oily** • You tan easily • Your skin tone is olive to dark • Your skin breaks out frequently • Your skin is highly elastic • You have blackheads and enlarged pores • Your skin looks shiny an hour after cleansing • As you get older, you will have few facial lines **Dry** • Your skin tends to burn, and peels soon after • Your skin gets itchy and irritated, especially in the winter • Your cheeks and forehead get dry and chapped • Your face feels tight after cleansing • Your complexion is fair **Sensitive** • Your skin burns quickly in the sun • You are fair-skinned • Certain ingredients cause your skin to burn or redden • You flush easily and often • Your skin is dry, fragile, and translucent • You have rough, scaly patches • Your face feels tight after cleansing • You have allergic reactions to certain ingredients and fragrances **Older** • Your skin burns easily • Your skin has allergic reactions to things it could support before • Your skin is fragile and shows everything more • You flush easily • Your skin is inelastic • Your skin rarely breaks out • Your pores are enlarged • You have deepening lines around your eyes, mouth, and forehead • Your complexion looks dull • You have broken capillaries on your cheeks or nose • Your skin is getting drier

SKIN TYPE

faQ **What is the T-zone?** The T-zone consists of your forehead, nose, and chin. For many people, it's the first place on the face that gets oily.

33

NORMAL SKIN IS SMOOTH AND SUPPLE, AND SUFFERS RELATIVELY FEW BREAKOUTS. IT IS NOT KNOWN AS "NORMAL" BECAUSE IT IS MORE COMMON THAN OILY OR DRY SKIN. NEITHER TOO OILY NOR TOO DRY,

it is skin that exists in balance—and what could be *less* common than that? It benefits from having a high natural water content in the outermost layer, a healthy natural lipid film to lock in moisture and prevent evaporation, and an efficient means of drawing moisture up from the dermis to the surface of the skin. That doesn't mean that normal skin is always well behaved. "Combination" skin is, essentially, normal skin on a bender. It can be oily, especially in the T-zone. It can be dry, especially in winter. It can be sensitive to environmental factors, like sun, cold, and pollution. The most important thing to realize about normal skin is that it's a rare gift.

 Normal skin does pretty well on its own. Your job is to find a regimen that doesn't interfere with your body's natural balance, but lends a hand when needed. A healthy diet, exercise regimen, and sleep schedule are all-important. A gentle **CLEANSER** for daily washing, a light day **MOISTURIZER** (heavier in colder climates) with SPF, and occasional use of a nonstripping **TONER** make up the bulk of what you'll need. **BREAKOUTS** can be controlled spot by spot with over-the-counter solutions of benzoyl peroxide.

"The Lord prefers common-looking people. That is why he makes so many of them."

ABRAHAM LINCOLN

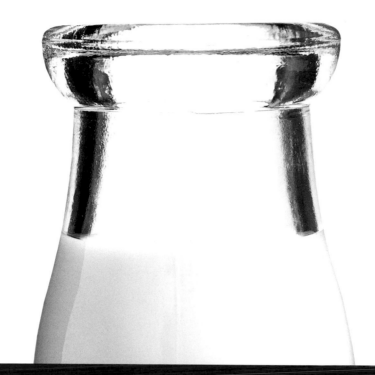
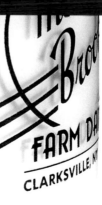

NORMAL

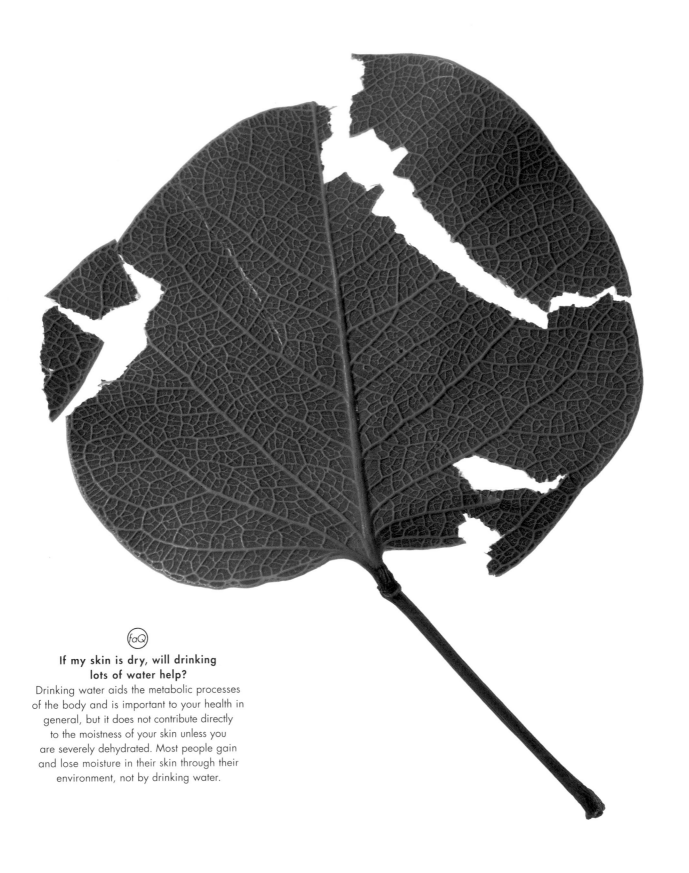

**If my skin is dry, will drinking
lots of water help?**

Drinking water aids the metabolic processes
of the body and is important to your health in
general, but it does not contribute directly
to the moistness of your skin unless you
are severely dehydrated. Most people gain
and lose moisture in their skin through their
environment, not by drinking water.

DRY

ITCHY, SCALY, CHAPPED, SORE—NONE OF THEM ARE TERMS WE WANT TO USE TO DESCRIBE THE WAY OUR SKIN FEELS, BUT THESE ARE THE PROPERTIES OF A DRY COMPLEXION. IT IS THE MOST COMMON OF SKIN

afflictions—not just a specific skin type but a reaction many of us experience periodically throughout our lives. Dry skin crosses all complexion boundaries, though it is especially common in those with fairer skin tones and is one symptom of sensitive skin in general. Many factors cause dehydration, among them certain medications, air travel, changes of season, chlorine, and hot water from bathing. The simple process of getting older makes our skin dry as well. But dry skin is not dry solely due to lack of oil or moisture. It results in part from shedding epidermal skin cells in clumps instead of cell by cell. One thing you can't blame on dry skin is wrinkles. They will show up more in a dry complexion, but you can't moisturize away environmental factors, which are the true culprits.

HOW TO **MAKEUP.** Moisturizing foundations and powders have a higher oil content, as do tinted moisturizers. **CLEANSER.** Lotion and milk cleansers are more moisturizing than gels, which can further dry your face, and soaps, which are out of the question. Long, hot showers and baths exacerbate dry skin problems. Use lukewarm water, pat yourself dry afterward, then apply moisturizer to lock in the thin layer of water still on your skin. **TONER.** Stay away from alcohol-based astringents. Look for a toner that has been especially formulated for dry skin. **MOISTURIZERS.** Look for heavier creams, especially for cold weather and night care, but be sure that they won't clog your pores or inhibit the shedding of dead skin cells. Humectants like lactic acid can also be useful in loosening scaly skin. Humidifiers and a slightly heavier night cream can help fight dry skin, especially in winter. There are also extraemollient spot treatments available for particularly dry patches: dab them on before applying moisturizer. **EXFOLIATORS.** Gentle exfoliating with a fine scrub or an AHA (alpha-hydroxy acid) lotion once a week may help skin absorb moisturizer better, but be careful: your skin may be too sensitive even for very light solutions.

[WRINKLES *first aid—page 174*]

O I L Y

BREAKOUTS ARE SUPPOSED TO STOP AFTER OUR TEENS, RIGHT? WRONG. MORE THAN 60 PERCENT OF WOMEN CONTINUE TO GET PIMPLES AND BLACKHEADS INTO THEIR THIRTIES AND FORTIES. THOSE WITH

darker and olive skin tones suffer more—though they don't burn in the sun and tend to wrinkle less. The chief culprit is overactive sebaceous glands. Pores become enlarged. A greasy shine appears on the chin, nose, and forehead. The surface of the skin can be coarse and lack elasticity. The temptation is to overclean, using harsh astringents, but this just makes the glands produce more oil. Start within. Alcohol, caffeine, spices, and foods containing iodides, like shellfish, can sometimes stimulate oil production. Don't touch your face, and don't exercise while you're wearing foundation or moisturizer.

HOW TO

CLEANSER. Use a mild cleanser to wash your face twice a day, but do not scrub away natural oils that your skin needs for protection. Gel cleansers clean gently without leaving a residue. **TONER.** Alcohol-based astringents are ideal for wiping away leftover residue from cleansers and excess oil between cleansings. **MOISTURIZER.** Look for lighter, noncomedogenic (does not clog pores) or nonacnegenic (does not irritate pores) formulations made especially for oily skin. Humectants can help soothe scaly reactions to acne medications. **EXFOLIATORS.** Gentle exfoliating may help keep skin clean and absorbent, so that minimal amounts of moisturizer can be used to maximum effect. Retin-A and Renova, as well as gentle AHA peels, can help certain acne-related problems. **MAKEUP.** Look for oil-free foundation, powder, and blush, as well as noncomedogenic and nonacnegenic makeup. Powder blush is less likely to aggravate acne than cream or gel.

BREAKOUTS. Minor breakouts can be controlled with over-the-counter solutions of benzoyl peroxide. Dermatologists treat more serious conditions with more serious solutions. Oral antibiotics, like tetracycline and erythromycin, attack pore-clogging bacteria and are available in topical form as well. Retin-A short-circuits pimple production by unclogging follicles below the surface of the skin. More holistic approaches combine gentle cleansing routines using potent plant extracts like apple, cucumber, and tea-tree oils, proper nutrition, and exercise to help fight unruly skin. **BLACK SKIN.** It can seem shiny and does not have the same problems with dryness as lighter skin, but that doesn't always mean black skin is oily. It reflects the light differently, giving off a kind of luminosity. Don't try to remove oil with harsh astringents. Cleanse and moisturize with gentle products geared to your skin type. Excess shine can be controlled by using oil-free bases and powder.

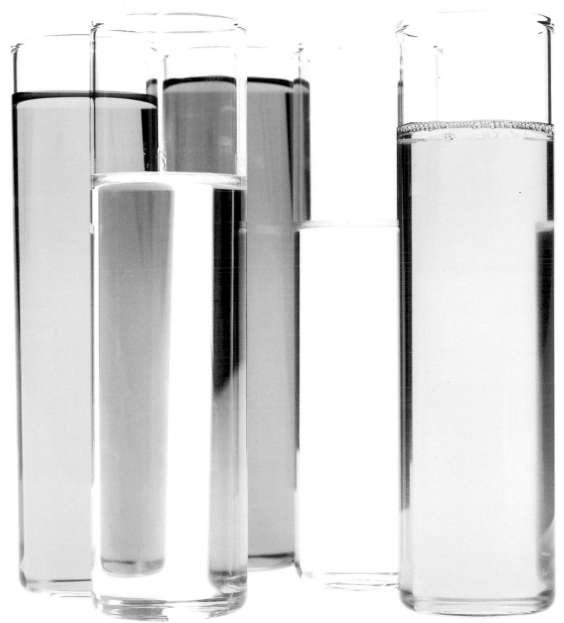

How can I clear up blackheads? Regular deep-cleaning facials clean out your pores—and, unfortunately, your pocketbook. Over-the-counter salycylic acid solutions, like the ones found in certain astringents and acne medications, can help. So can creams containing benzoyl peroxide, which kills bacteria. Retin-A clears blackheads on top of treating acne by unclogging pores. Light exfoliation twice a week will also help to keep pores clean.

Due to hormonal fluctuations, your skin will be oilier when you're premenstrual.

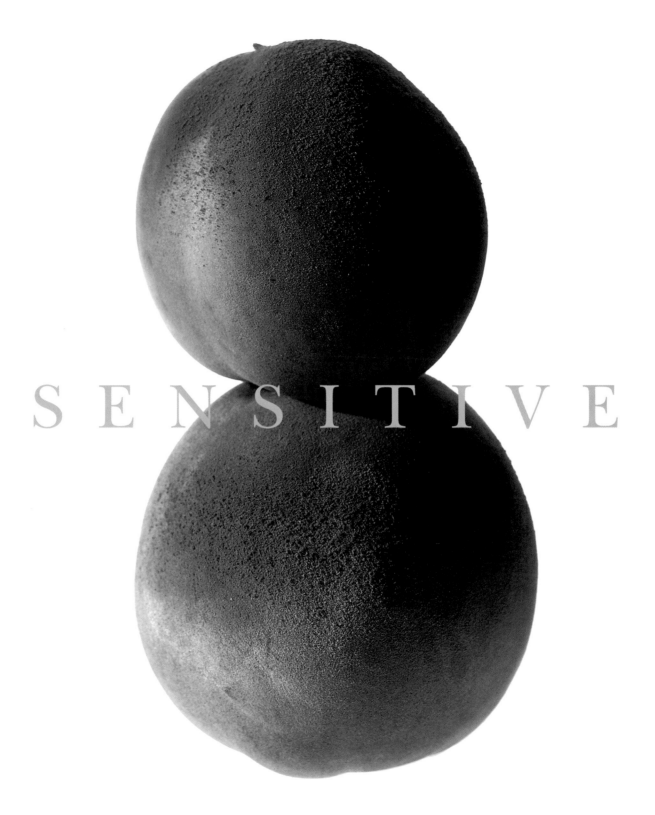

TRULY SENSITIVE SKIN IS RARE. A RECENT STUDY FOUND THAT WHILE 60 PERCENT OF US BELIEVE OUR SKIN IS SENSITIVE, THE ACTUAL NUMBER MAY BE CLOSER TO 6 PERCENT. WE TEND TO HAVE FAIR COMPLEXIONS.

Our skin is pale and thin. We blush purple at the drop of a hat. We burn under a 40-watt bulb. We have allergic reactions to food, pollen, soap, and, of course, to the very products we use to soothe ourselves. Our faces get blotchy and covered in dry, flaky patches. We are particularly susceptible to conditions like rosacea and couperose, in which spidery red capillaries and sometimes small, red, acnelike bumps appear on the surface of the skin. The cause of all this misery? A weak protective lipid barrier. The epidermis contains dead cells and fatty molecules called lipids, which help lock in moisture and protect against pollution, temperature extremes, sun, and other environmental hazards. Any product—scrubs, AHAs, tretinoin (the active ingredient in Retin-A and Renova)— that breaks down the barrier function by helping us exfoliate also runs the risk of making us more sensitive to whatever we put on immediately afterward. Avoid experimenting with a variety of products at once—your skin may have an adverse reaction. Try one product at a time and add others gradually to isolate problems easily.

HOW TO The world is full of things for us to avoid. Products with fragrance, fruit acids, exfoliating enzymes, irritating vitamins, and plant extracts. Certain preservatives, like BHA, Quaternium-15, and Bronopol, might cause problems as well. **CLEANSER.** Very mild lotion or milk cleansers. No stripping gels or drying soaps. Tepid water and nothing abrasive, like scratchy washcloths or scrubs. Products containing chamomile and jojoba can be soothing. **TONERS.** If any, then nonalcoholic toners especially formulated for sensitive skin—look for rosewater, orangewater, or witch hazel. **MOISTURIZER.** Again, hypoallergenic and fragrance-free, with as few ingredients as possible. Remember: the purer the product, the less likely you are to be allergic to it. **EXFOLIATORS.** None. Sensitive skin needs to be treated with great care. **MAKEUP.** Hypoallergenic foundations and powders that are fragrance-free. Moisturizing products to counter sensitive skin's tendency to be dry.

[✹ SENSITIVE SKIN *first aid—page 173*]

41

Older

WE AGE. OUR CIRCULATORY SYSTEM PUMPS MORE SLOWLY, BRINGING LESS BLOOD TO OUR SKIN AND causing dehydration. We make fewer new cells, and the cells we do create lose their ability to adhere to one another. Melanocytes, which control pigmentation, become fewer and work less efficiently: we get blotchy or lose color. Collagen production slows down, making our skin less elastic. And that's just the natural aging process. Years of exposure to the sun gives us leathery, lined skin, as well as age spots, broken blood vessels, and scaly precancers known as actinic keratoses. Gravity pulls on us, causing the corners of our mouths to turn down and eyelids and chins to droop. Facial expressions we have had over the decades and lines that form when we sleep in certain positions become permanently etched in our skin. A lifetime of hormonal changes begins to take its toll. The result is skin that may sometimes look crepey, dry, wrinkled, blotchy, dull, or irritated.

MENOPAUSE AND THE SKIN. Estrogen keeps the skin supple and well hydrated. During menopause, estrogen levels are reduced by half, or even two-thirds, while testosterone decreases only slightly. The loss of estrogen causes the skin to become thinner and less supple, so that it becomes duller and less light-reflective. The relatively high level of testosterone can result in increased facial hair and larger sebaceous glands and pores. It also can contribute to breakouts by thickening the oils that naturally occur on the face and slowing down exfoliation.

HOW TO Treat older skin gently and with respect. Eat right and exercise. Coddle new sensitivities with **CLEANSERS** that are gentle and nondrying. Steer clear of soap and alcohol-based products. **MOISTURIZE** with a light, readily absorbed day cream with an SPF. At night, take special care around the eyes and upper lip, and use a heavier moisturizer. If it does not irritate your skin, gentle **EXFOLIATING**—with a scrub or a light acid formula like an AHA moisturizer—can slough off dead cells and allow your moisturizer to penetrate more easily. Tretinoin solutions like Retin-A and Renova may make your skin look smoother and less lined, but they can be irritating. **MAKEUP** should incorporate moisturizing formulas. It should also not be too heavy, or it will call attention to wrinkles.

[WRINKLES *first aid—page 174*]

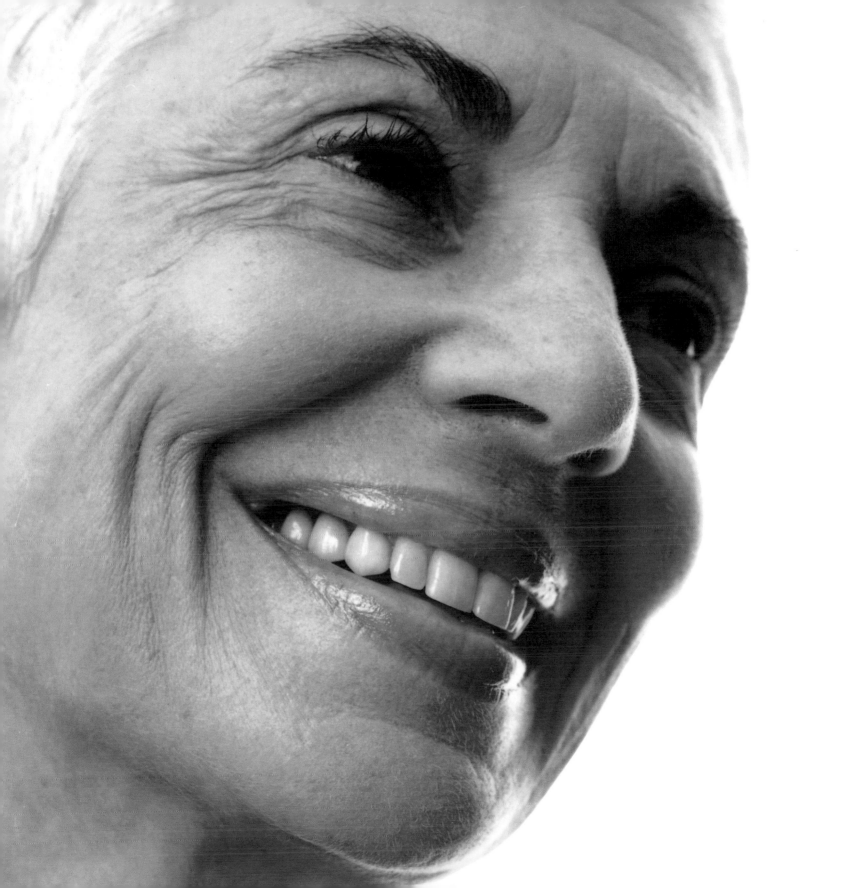

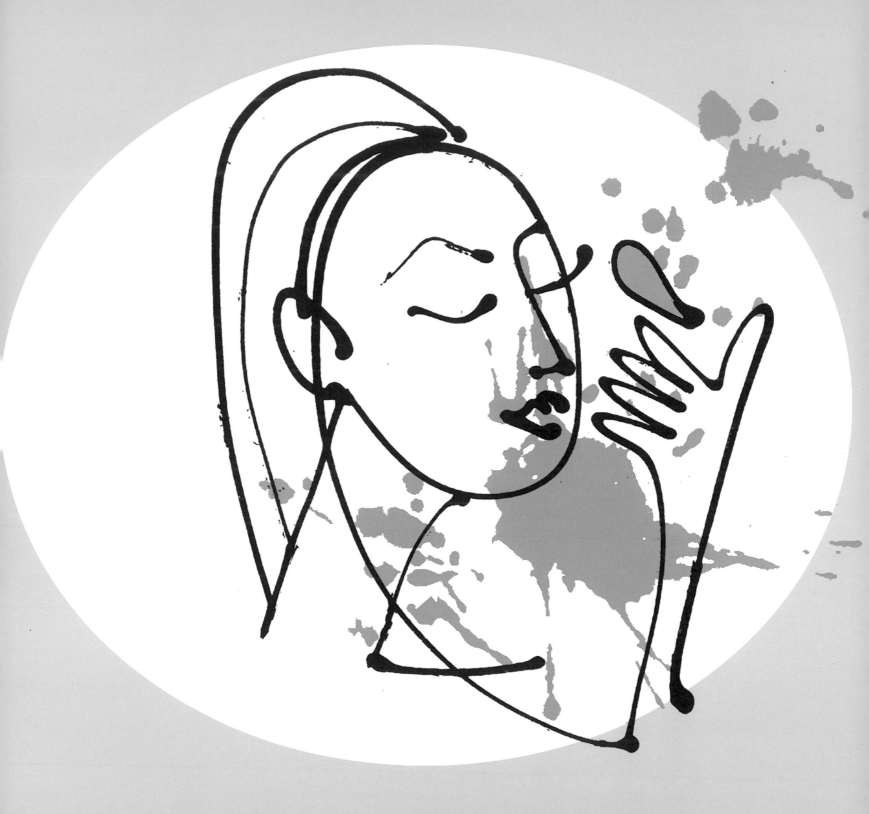

CHAPTER 3

Taking Care of Your Skin

What's the best way to clean my skin? [page 50]   Do I have to use a different cleanser to remove eye makeup? [page 49]

Are toners really necessary? [page 52]

What kind of facial mask is right for me? [page 55]

Do I need a different moisturizer at night? [page 58]

How should I apply moisturizer? [page 59]

"Well-groomed people are the real beauties. It doesn't matter what they're wearing or who they're with or how much their jewelry costs or how much their clothes cost or how perfect their makeup is: **if they're not clean, they're not beautiful."**

ANDY WARHOL, *The Philosophy of Andy Warhol*

S K I N C A R E

Clean. Moisturize. Protect. The Three Commandments of basic skin care. As with any rule, you'll want to break one of them once in a while. Try not to. They work as a package even as they apply differently to each one of us, depending on our age and skin type. As usual, there is always more you can do for better results. You can soothe, deep-clean, or deep-moisturize your skin with facial masks. You can slough off dead skin cells—gently, please—with exfoliants. You can dot your blemishes with drying solutions. Or you can simply clean, moisturize, and protect your skin every day. You're the boss.

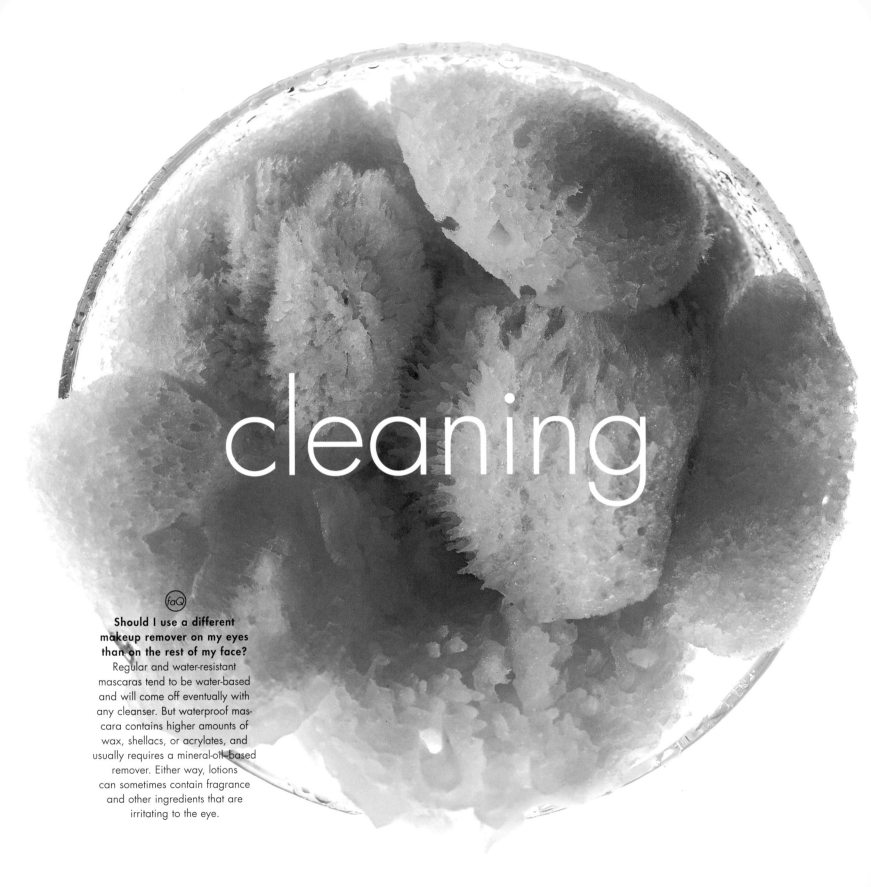

cleaning

Should I use a different makeup remover on my eyes than on the rest of my face?
Regular and water-resistant mascaras tend to be water-based and will come off eventually with any cleanser. But waterproof mascara contains higher amounts of wax, shellacs, or acrylates, and usually requires a mineral-oil–based remover. Either way, lotions can sometimes contain fragrance and other ingredients that are irritating to the eye.

SQUEAKY CLEAN

IT'S A TIME-HONORED SENSUAL RITUAL: THE SMELL OF CLEANSER. THE SOUND OF SPLASHING. THE FEEL OF A CLEAN, DRY TOWEL. WAS IT EVER AS SIMPLE AS SOAP AND WATER? CLEARLY, RENAISSANCE WOMEN who washed their faces in their own urine didn't think so. How and with what you cleanse your skin depends on your skin type. Vary your cleaning routine according to changes in weather and climate. Harsh winds and cold demand gentle treatment. Tropical humidity may require a more rigorous approach.

HOW TO REMOVE YOUR MAKEUP. Before you clean your skin, you need to take off your makeup with lotion and eye-makeup remover. Makeup is a creamy substance and needs to be dissolved with an oil-based cream before you wash, no matter what your skin type. Those with sensitive complexions should avoid heavily fragranced products. Special makeup-removing lotions exist, but in a pinch any moisturizer will do—especially if the alternative is ducking under the covers with a fully made-up face. Wearing makeup to bed can clog your pores, and mascara can break your lashes. **EYES:** Take off eye makeup first. Clean gently until the cotton pad comes away clean. Clean residue under lower lid by wiping from the outside to the inside corner of the eye. Blot oily film away gently with a tissue. Never pull or rub the fragile skin around the eye. **FACE:** Apply cleansing lotion or regular moisturizing cream to a clean, damp cotton pad to clean jawline, cheek area, and underneath the eye, wiping in upward horizontal strokes to the ear. Take a clean pad and clean the forehead from temple to temple. Use a fresh cotton pad and a new dab of lotion to wipe down your nose and around each nostril. Finally, use a clean pad to wipe lipstick from one side to the other, then turn the pad over and wipe in the opposite direction. Blot residue with a tissue. If you wear a lot of makeup, repeat the entire process. Follow your normal cleansing routine to wash away any greasy film.

Cleansers

Foaming cleansers contain surfactants—molecules that dissolve oil-based materials on the skin. They are gentle enough for **NORMAL SKIN** but strong enough to handle the oilier T-zone. Water and oil don't mix, which is why we can't depend on H_2O alone to penetrate greasy buildup on the surface of our skin. Gels are virtually oil free. Less alkaline than soap,

> "You can do whatever you want and if you're not happy, go to the bathroom, wash your face, and you become yourself again."
>
> STÉPHANE MARAIS

they rinse off easily, even in cold water, and leave virtually no residue. They are good for **OILY** and **NORMAL SKIN**. Sometimes foaming cleansers and gels can be too harsh. Lotions contain milder surfactants and a moisturizer and are good for **DRY SKIN**. Emollient-rich cream cleansers leave a light film to soothe dry skin. Be sure to wash off creams with a warm, wet washcloth or sponge to avoid pore-clogging residue.

HOW TO CLEAN YOUR SKIN. Start with warm water, the right cleanser for your skin type, and either a washcloth, a sponge, or your hands. Wet your skin with tepid water, then rub the cleanser between your palms to warm it up (it will spread and absorb dirt better). Gently massage the cleanser over your entire face, paying special attention to oily areas like the nose, chin, and forehead. Do not scrub. Rinse the cleanser off with a washcloth, a sponge, or your hands, treating your face sensitively (a washcloth is a gentle way to exfoliate). Blot with a clean towel. If your skin feels soft ten to fifteen minutes after cleansing, you're using the right stuff. If it still feels tight, then you may be using a cleanser that's stripping away too much oil. Overcleaning oily skin leads to an increase in oil production. To avoid drying out skin by overcleaning, cleanse skin thoroughly at night only. Each morning, rinse with cool water or a toner if you feel the need to clean and refresh. For extra-deep cleaning, use an exfoliant or a cleansing mask. Sensitive skin may be able to withstand such treatment only once a month, while oilier skin may benefit from it weekly.

SOAP STORY

Soap is generally made from animal fats, vegetable oils, and some form of alkali salt. It breaks down to absorb dirt and oil, surrounding them with a protective colloid that prevents reabsorption. Moisturizing soaps tend to be less alkaline, owing to added citric or lactic acid, and are therefore less irritating. Sulfur, salicylic acid, and benzoyl peroxide soaps reduce oiliness, benefiting acne-prone skin. Soap for sensitive skin is super-fatted, which means that a moisturizer like cold cream, lanolin, olive oil, or cocoa butter has been added. Normal soaps contain less than 2 percent fat. Superfatted formulas usually contain between 5 and 15 percent fat. Transparent soaps are a form of superfatted soap, containing glycerin, alcohol, and sugar. Energizing soaps often contain mild abrasives, like salicylic acid. Or they may simply have extracts that make your skin tingle, like peppermint or lavender.

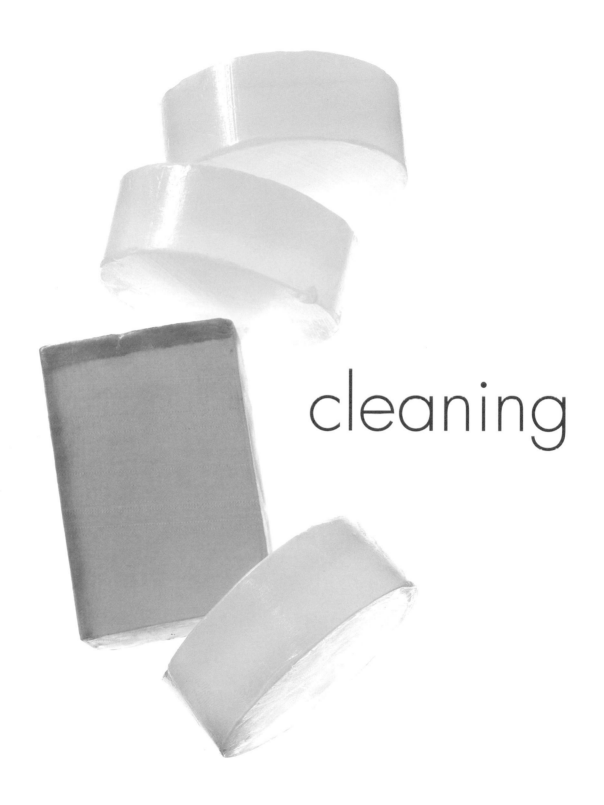

cleaning

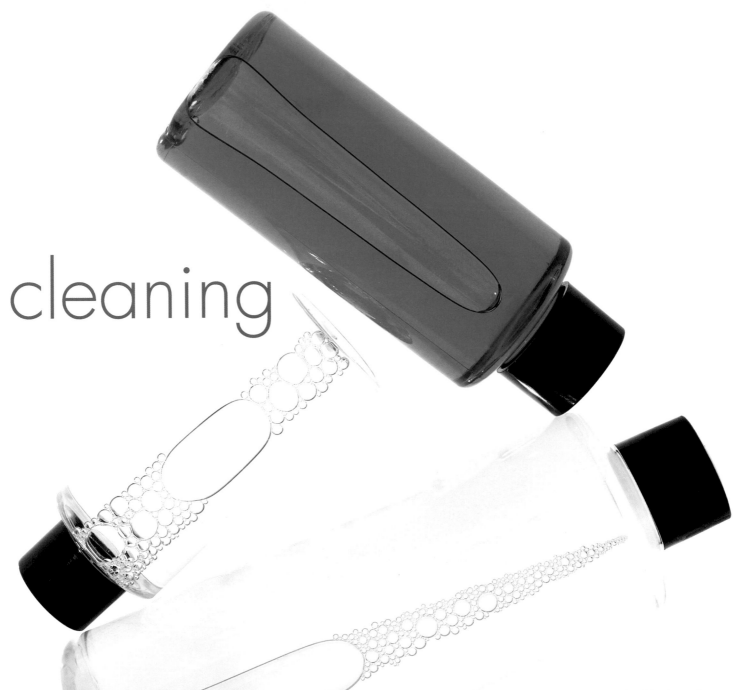

cleaning

TONERS, ASTRINGENTS, AND CLARIFYING LOTIONS. All three remove dirt and oil, but some do it more harshly than others. Astringents and clarifying lotions containing alcohol are most efficient for removing greasy buildup from oily and acne-prone skin. They can be drying and should not be overused. Good toners aren't drying for normal skin, but sensitive and dry complexions may want to avoid even the milder alcohol-free formulations. Some toners do come specially formulated for sensitive skin and can be useful for cleaning or freshening between cleansings.

[🧊 PIMPLES *first aid—page 173*]

extra clean

SIMPLE CLEANING WITH WARM WATER AND A FACIAL CLEANSER IS THE IMPORTANT PART, BUT EVERY ONCE IN A WHILE IT'S ALSO A GOOD IDEA TO TREAT YOUR FACE TO A LITTLE EXTRA. IT COULD BE A SCRUB, OR TONER, OR A PROFESSIONAL FACIAL. JUST BE SURE TO KEEP YOUR SKIN TYPE IN MIND TO AVOID OVERDOING IT.

Exfoliants. Although it is the outer limit of our protection against the harsh realities of weather, pollution, and the sun, the bricklike formation of our outer-skin cells can feel scaly and dry. It can also inhibit the absorption of moisture and protective barriers, like moisturizing creams and lotions. It can contribute to the appearance of dull, dead-looking skin. And it can prevent makeup from covering smoothly. What to do? Slough it off.

Scrubs. Although they vary in consistency, scrubs are usually lotions or creams containing rough particles like sand, pumice, or crushed fruit pits. They tend to combine a soothing moisturizer with the relatively abrasive sandpaper approach to removing dead skin. Exfoliating can cause broken capillaries and irritation in sensitive skin.

Alpha-Hydroxy Acids. Cleopatra, who was reputed to bathe in a mixture of lemon juice and donkey's milk, knew all about AHAs. They occur naturally in unripened fruit, but most are manufactured synthetically to mimic natural substances. They include a range of acids, among them glycolic acid (sugar cane), malic acid (apples), tartaric acid (grapes), and citric acid (citrus and molasses). Fruit acids dissolve the intracellular cement —a gluelike substance that holds together the outer layer of skin—allowing for a more rapid exfoliation. In theory, this should result in fresher-looking skin, but the effectiveness of AHAs has recently been disputed by the FDA. You can find them in over-the-counter solutions—typically under 5-percent concentration—but doctors often prescribe solutions between 12- and 15-percent concentration.

Tretinoin. Used for decades as an acne treatment, prescription formulas of vitamin-A–derived solutions like Retin-A and Renova have been found to have a variety of beneficial effects on sun-damaged, aging skin. On the surface, they exfoliate by dissolving the top layer of skin. But under the surface of the skin, they have been found to increase collagen and elastin production, increase the formation of new blood vessels, restore the epidermis to a thicker, healthier, more evenly pigmented state, and even reverse certain precancerous lesions. The result? Rosier, smoother, less wrinkled skin. Now for the bad news: tretinoin solutions can be irritating to sensitive and dry skin. They should be used sparingly, only where needed, and applied at least twenty minutes after cleansing, when the skin has dried thoroughly. They should be used in concert with very gentle cleansers and moisturizers, to reduce skin irritation. And because they increase sun sensitivity, you should stay well protected from indirect sunlight and completely out of direct sunlight.

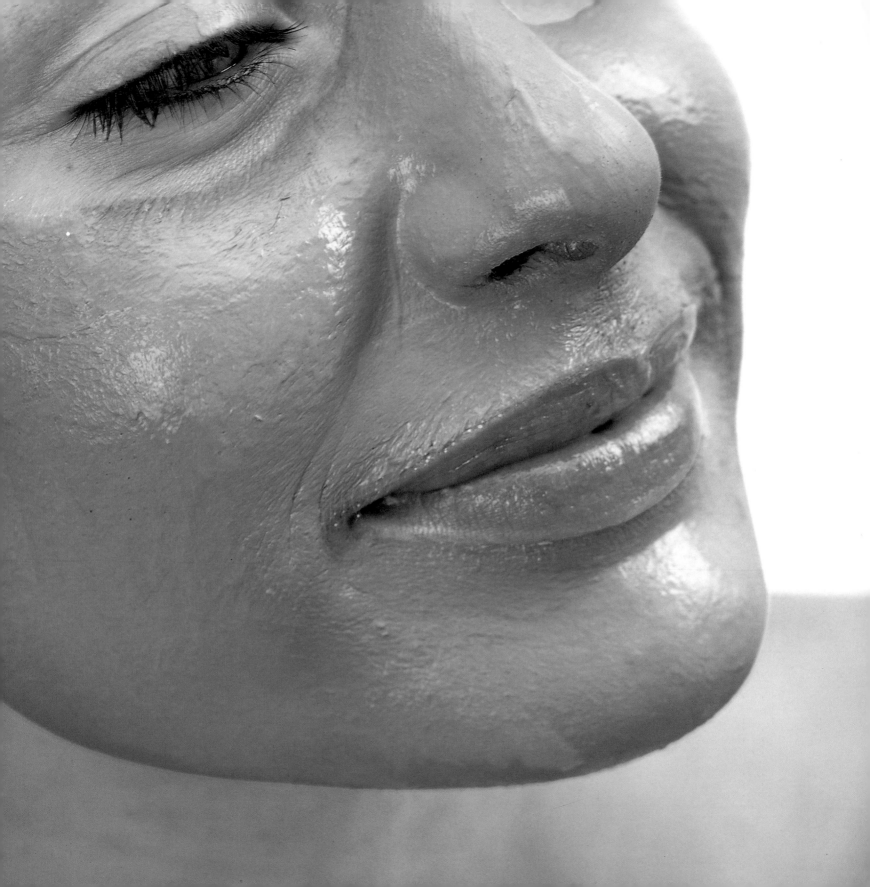

M A S K S

OUR MOTHERS MAY AS WELL HAVE BEEN CASTING THEIR FACES IN CEMENT. MASKS WENT ON THICK AND COLD, AND DRIED HARD AND FAST. TODAY'S MASKS CAN BE WET OR DRY, AND TREAT A RANGE OF ILLS.

OILY OR BROKEN-OUT SKIN. Deep-cleansing clay or mud masks soak up oil, draw out impurities, and tighten pores. Antibacterial agents help subdue hot spots. Corn or wheat starch, charcoal, or titanium dioxide in the mask helps boost oil dry-up. This mask can be applied over the entire face, or just over the T-zone. **DRY SKIN.** Moisturizing masks bring a mixture of moisture and nutrients—essential fatty acids, vegetable proteins, amino acids, hyaluronic acid, urea, and algae—to parched skin. The cream or gel base provides a barrier to help skin hang on to its own natural moisture. **IRRITATED OR SENSITIVE SKIN.** A gel or cream-based mask with soothing anti-inflammatory ingredients like algae, azulene, or chamomile delivers immediate relief. A gel is best for oily or sensitive skin. A cream-based mask works better for dry skin. **NORMAL OR DULL SKIN.** A sloughing mask helps exfoliate dead skin that can result from pollution, stress, airplane flights, or sun exposure. Use a cream for gentler sloughing action on more sensitive skin, a peel-off AHA mask for normal skin.

FACIALS. Do they really help your skin over the long haul? As usual, there are two sides to the story. Dermatologists say the deep-cleaning effects of a facial last a scant few days, though they admit that cleaning out pores is good for your skin. Facialists argue that a monthly facial is important for getting rid of the dead cells that accumulate in the natural cycle of skin growth. Most facials involve several steps: analysis of the skin; steaming to open pores; deep cleaning through extraction; massage; application of at least one mask or light peel; and hydration with an appropriate moisturizer. Facials usually take about one hour, and can cost between $50 and $100. Mention any medication you're using, especially Accutane or Retin-A—you should be careful about using any AHA products on top of these treatments. Stay away from facials during your period, when your skin is especially sensitive. Take out contact lenses to avoid smearing and eye irritation. Keep your face free of makeup for a few hours after the facial to allow skin to breathe. Don't be surprised if all that poking and squeezing leads to a breakout or two in the days following your facial.

Moisturize

MOISTURIZERS DO NOT MOISTURIZE. THEY SMOOTH AND SOFTEN YOUR SKIN BY CREATING A BARRIER THAT REPLACES NATURAL OILS AND LOCKS IN MOISTURE ABSORBED BY WASHING. THEY CAN ALSO SOMETIMES

provide relief from itchy, irritated skin. They are concocted from a combination of occlusive ingredients (animal fats, vegetable or mineral oils, or silicone oil derivatives) and humectants (glycerin, propylene glycol, butylene glycol, urea, lactic acid, or lecithin), which draw water up from the lower levels of the dermis to the outer "horny layer" of the epidermis. They differ widely not only in the types of oil they contain but also in their proportions of oil and water. Some of them, like lanolin and cocoa butter, are potentially more irritating and acne-provoking than others.

Apply moisturizer to damp skin immediately after cleansing your face. This allows the product to replace any natural oils you've cleaned away and locks in water that has been absorbed by washing. **NORMAL SKIN.** You may not need a moisturizer, but if you do, try a light, water-based, hypoallergenic lotion. **DRY SKIN.** Oil-based moisturizers can be good for dry skin, especially if they contain a powerful humectant like urea. **OILY OR ACNE-PRONE SKIN.** You may not need a moisturizer, especially if you live in a warm climate, although some acne treatments can be drying. Look for moisturizers that are noncomedogenic or nonacnegenic, which will reduce pore clogging. Silicone moisturizers are oil-free and are best for acne-prone skin. Avoid ingredients like isopropyl myristate, isopropyl esters, oleic acid, stearic acid, lanolin, heavy mineral oil, linseed oil, olive oil, and cocoa butter. **COMBINATION SKIN.** Remember that moisturizers do not have brains and therefore cannot treat different parts of your face differently. You may need to treat oily patches with one product and dry patches with another. **SENSITIVE SKIN.** Find a product with as few ingredients as possible to cut down your chances of irritation. Try spot-testing a light, fragrance-free, hypoallergenic moisturizer for a few days.

Wait at least ten minutes between applying your moisturizer and your makeup (blot with a tissue if you're uncertain). Otherwise, your makeup could run or disappear entirely.

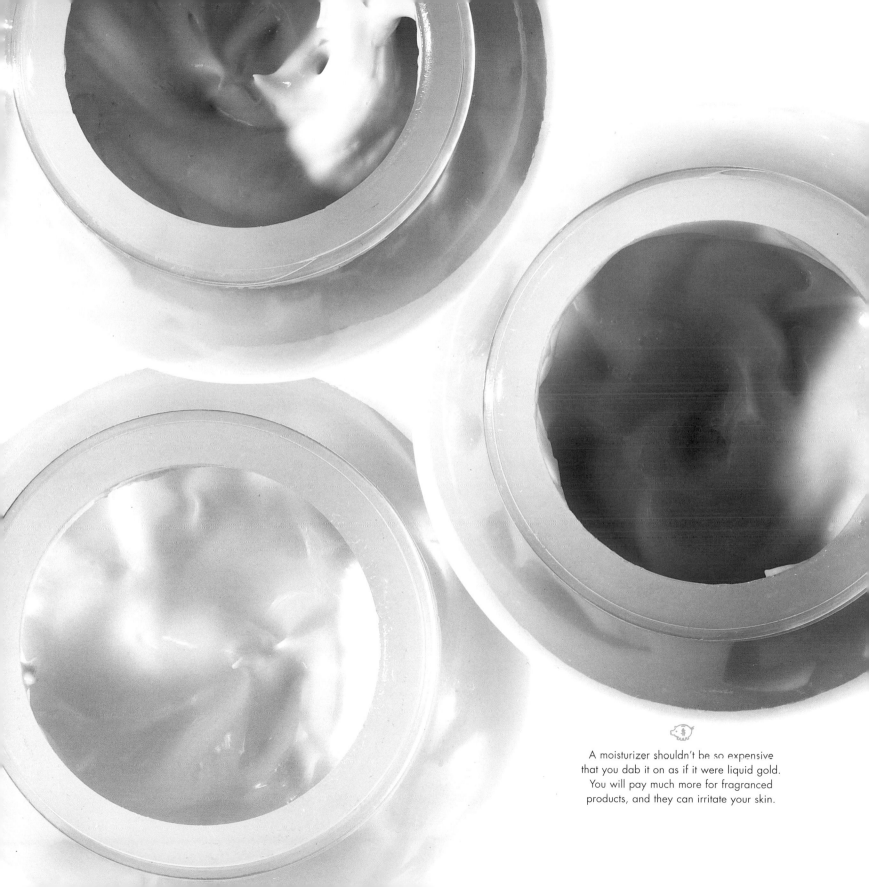

A moisturizer shouldn't be so expensive
that you dab it on as if it were liquid gold.
You will pay much more for fragranced
products, and they can irritate your skin.

Moisturize CONT'D.

Active moisture. An increasing number of moisturizers now come with active ingredients, such as AHAs and sunscreens. A few general rules: AHAs are said to improve the smoothness and appearance of your skin. A dermatologist can prescribe higher doses than you will be able to find in over-the-counter lotions. The downside to AHAs? They can be irritating to sensitive or dry skin. And they often smell funny. SPF moisturizers are an ideal way to ensure that you have at least some sun protection on your face. The only problem? Usually you do not slather on facial moisturizer thickly enough to provide any real guard against extended time in the sun. And sometimes SPFs can irritate sensitive skin. Shop around until you find a good SPF moisturizer with the right consistency. It's certainly better than having nothing at all, and more reliable than counting on an SPF foundation, which you will apply even more sparingly. **Eyes.** The skin around your eyes is more fragile than the skin elsewhere on your face, as it tends to be thinner and have fewer oil glands. Avoid harsh cleansers, and wash the eye area only in the evening, after you've removed your makeup. Natural ingredients like butcher's broom, marigold, and slippery elm can constrict blood vessels and reduce puffiness. Cucumber slices can be soothing to tired, irritated eyes. AHAs can help reduce fine lines. But most important of all, use an eye cream night and day for protection against weather, climate, and the sun. **Lips.** Like the skin around the eyes, the skin on your lips is very delicate. It contains fewer melanin cells, so it burns easily. And it is thin, so it wrinkles, chaps, and peels more frequently than the rest of your face. Apply a protective lip balm regularly. It can double as a gloss or tone down a dark lip color. **Night and Day.** Thick, heavy, shiny night creams offer heavy-duty moisturizing that an invisible day formulation can't possibly match. They can make a mess of your pillowcase if you're not used to sleeping on your back, though. And if, for some reason, you want to wear a night moisturizer in the daytime, don't do it—at least not outdoors: the nighttime varieties aren't formulated with sun protection.

☼ If you're not happy with the way a moisturizer feels on your face, use it on your hands instead.

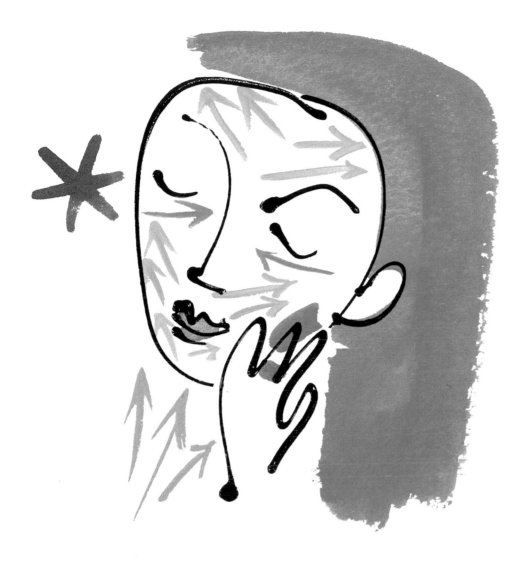

 Because gravity pulls your skin down, massage moisturizer into your face and neck with upward-moving gestures. First dot eye moisturizer over the delicate skin around each eye, moving inward and upward but never rubbing hard. Then apply facial moisturizer by starting at the base of your neck, and rub cream up to the edge of your jawline. From the center of your chin, move your fingertips up and out, always working wrinkles in the opposite direction. Finally, from the center of your forehead, work moisturizer out and up, toward your hairline.

Delicate skin around the eyes can be protected with a concentrated eye cream. A slightly heavier night cream, especially during the winter months, may help keep your skin supple and soft.

"When a Paris-based research company polled 300 European women and asked them what they would take with them to Mars, the number-one choice was moisturizer—ahead of husbands."

TRACY YOUNG

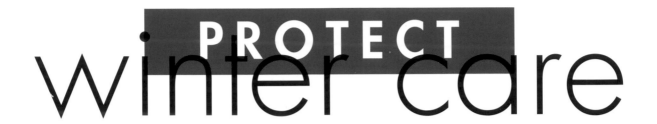

PROTECT winter care

WINTER SKIN IS ABOUT EXTREMES. WE LEAVE PARCHED, OVERHEATED ROOMS TO BATTLE FRIGID SNOW AND COLD, AND OUR SKIN PAYS THE PRICE. IT BECOMES RAW, CHAPPED, BLOTCHY, RED, ITCHY, AND

tight. In a word, it gets angry. The rules of winter: Protect and soothe. Avoid products with alcohol. Consider a more gentle cleansing routine, like using a mild milk cleanser with lukewarm water and a moisturizing mask to replenish and nourish irritated skin. Try specially formulated oils and lotions made from natural substances like lavender and rosewater to calm and heal. A heavier, non-water-based moisturizer can lock in moisture and protect against wind and cold. The delicate skin on your lips and eyes needs special attention. Use a lip balm and an eye cream day and night. Other tips? When outdoors, wrap a scarf around your face to protect sensitive capillaries from breaking. Wear sunglasses to protect your eyes, and to keep you from squinting (another cause of wrinkles). Fight dry indoor heat with humidifiers. Gently exfoliate dead cells to allow the skin to breathe and regenerate. And just because it's 20 below, don't forget to put on a sunscreen: snow and ice reflect harmful UV rays.

FROSTBITE. If you spend a lot of time outside in the winter—on the ski slopes, or skating, or working—beware of water-based moisturizers. They can actually freeze on, and into, your face, causing your skin severe distress. Oil-based moisturizers have a higher freezing point, and are therefore better for those cold months. Even for those with oily complexions, they shouldn't cause breakouts if they're used only occasionally.

[🗋 THE SEASONS *first aid—page 170*]

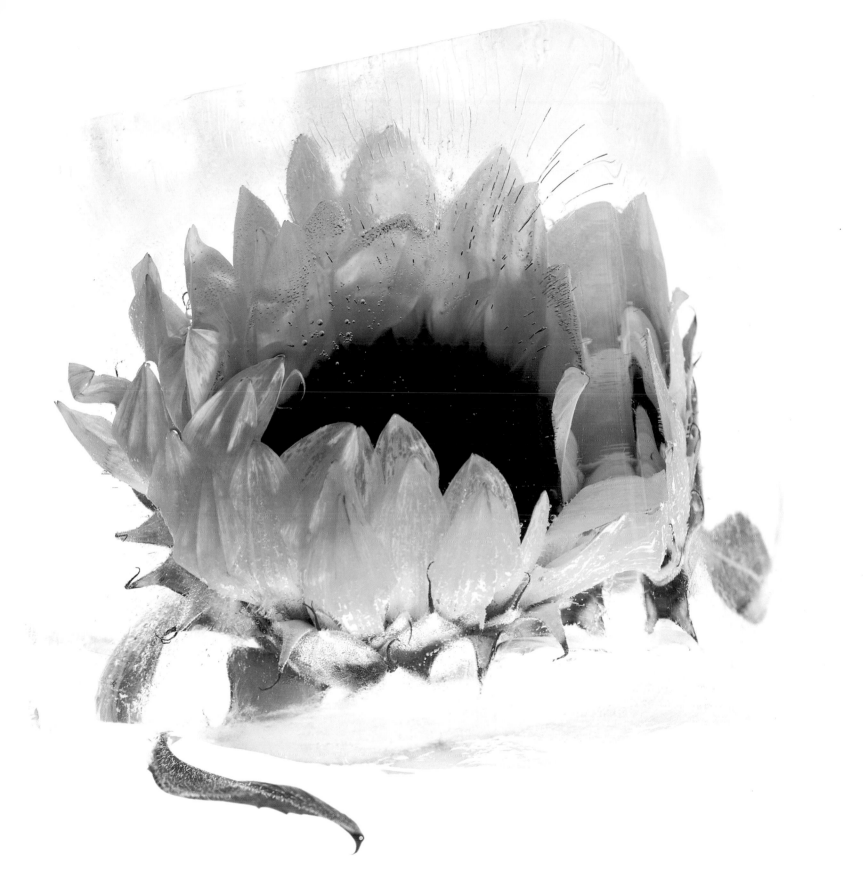

UVA and UVB

rays. Ultraviolet rays cause our
skin to burn and age. Both UVA and UVB rays
penetrate the epidermis and trigger melanin production.
Most sunscreens provide protection from UVB, which tends to
vary in intensity according to season, altitude, and time of day. UVA
rays ("aging rays") are more constant and harder to protect against. They
can burn through windows and loose-knit clothing to penetrate to the dermis, or
second layer of the skin, and affect collagen production.

Sunscreens.

Sunscreens do not prevent skin cancer. In fact, by providing
us with a sense of security, they can even do harm by increasing the amount of time we
allow ourselves to spend in the sun. Still, they are better than no protection at all. If your skin
burns easily, don't fool around with low-SPF formulas. Head straight for the sunblock—at least
SPF 15. SPF also indicates UVB absorption. SPF 15 absorbs 93 percent of UVB rays, while SPF
34 uses three times as many chemicals and delivers only 4 percent more absorption.

Sunscreens in makeup and moisturizers.

Titanium dioxide, a prime ingredient in many sunscreens, has been used to make cosmetics
more opaque since the 1970s, long before its protective qualities were known. And the FDA
does require SPF makeup to be subjected to the same tests as SPF sun lotions. This is just as
well, since you need all the protection you can get. Extra sunscreen in bases and moisturizers can never be a bad thing—just be sure to put enough on. And don't rely on a thin
coat of makeup for all your sun protection—layer it over a proper amount of SPF moisturizer. But remember that the numbers don't necessarily add up: an SPF 8 foundation
over an SPF 8 moisturizer does not mean a total SPF of 16. If you're afraid of too
much sunscreen buildup, get your SPF from your sunscreen alone.
Be sure you always put it on before going out.

Sunlamps.

Tanning parlors are perfectly safe if you
wear a hat and sunglasses and apply plenty of SPF 15 sunblock,
and stay away from the lamp between 10 a.m.
and 4 p.m. In other words, avoid
them altogether.

PROTECT
summer care

WE'RE DRAWN TO BASK IN THE SUN'S GLOW, AND IT'S KILLING US. OUR SKIN IS THE BATTLEGROUND. FIFTY YEARS AGO, ONE IN THIRTY-FIVE HUNDRED PEOPLE HAD MALIGNANT MELANOMA. TODAY, ONE IN THIRTY-SIX DOES.

Exposure to ultraviolet rays stimulates melanin production, which is why we tan. It also encourages rogue electrons known as free radicals to demolish the lipids, proteins, and nucleic acids in our epidermis. And deeper down, sunlight damages collagen, the connective tissue that keeps our skin firm and elastic. Creams containing vitamins A and E bring antioxidants to the skin's surface to consume and expel certain free radicals. Our bodies make enzymes to counteract other damage. Still, the fact remains: you can blame 80 percent of the skin's visible aging on exposure to the sun. The best protection? Use an SPF 15 sunscreen made with oxybenzone, titanium dioxide, or Parsol 1789. Slather it on generously, and apply it to all exposed skin. Don't forget your lips, which lack a protective keratin layer and burn easily. Avoid the prime griddle hours of 10 a.m. to 4 p.m. Wear a hat, sunglasses, and tightly knit clothing. Best of all, stay in the shade.

Does sun exposure improve or worsen acne?

Ultraviolet light temporarily suppresses oil production in the sebaceous glands, so acne can appear to improve after exposure to the sun. But nine to twelve days later, your glands go into overdrive to make up for lost time, and your skin will get worse. The sun is generally so bad for your skin that you should never use sunbathing as a quick fix for pimples.

"I don't tan—I stroke!"

WOODY ALLEN, in *Play It Again, Sam*

"I fake it so real, I am beyond fake."

COURTNEY LOVE, *"Doll Parts"*

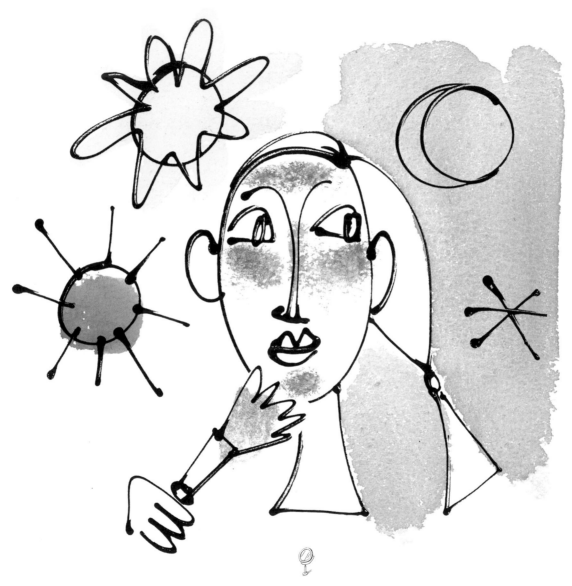

• Apply a bronzing powder all over your face with a large, soft brush. A little more can be used on the cheeks, nose, forehead, and chin.
• Try a soft, shimmery brown shadow applied to lids. • A little black mascara will give definition. • In the summer, lips look great when they're coated with a generous topping of tinted gloss. Warm, pink-brown tones create a natural look.

Fake It

WE SPENT CENTURIES INDOORS AND UNDER HATS. WE EVEN ATE ARSENIC TO AVOID LOOKING SUN-KISSED. NOW THAT WE CRAVE THE SUN, IT'S OFF LIMITS. BUT MANY OF US STILL LIKE TO LOOK AS IF WE'VE BEEN OUTDOORS, so we fake it with tanners. There are a few ground rules. Don't go more than two shades darker than your natural coloring—you'll look like you've been baked in a kiln. When you apply makeup over your artificial tan, transparent texture is the key. Use a sheer face tint, a tinted moisturizer, or a light, oil-free base. Or just use a light bronzing powder. You may be able to skip blush, but soft pinkish-bronze shades complement fair skin with a light tan. Darker skin tones can go deeper, but keep the color warm. Lips look best in sheer, glossy colors for summer.

HOW TO **TANNERS.** It's easy to go overboard: wait at least three hours to check your color before applying a second coat. Lightweight tanners are easier to spread and won't streak as much as thicker lotions. Generally, a fake tan will fade in two days unless you reapply your tanner every day—and be sure to wash your hands immediately after every application. AHA products will fade a fake tan because they exfoliate the very cells you have just colorized. **LIQUID AND CREME BRONZERS** are basically liquid foundations with a slight bronze color added, so you get some coverage along with your tan. They come in both oil-free and moisturizing formulas. **TINTED MOISTURIZERS** are more subtle in effect. They are perfect for fair skin that is dry, although they also come in oil-free formulas. **BRONZING STICKS** are quick and clean, but are not always as easy to blend well. **BRONZING POWDER** is the easiest and most popular route to a fake tan because it is light and can be applied over foundation if you need coverage. It comes in both loose and pressed form, and a wide range of colors. The trick is picking the right one for your skin tone. Stay with warm browns, not red-mahogany tones, and look for sheer textures.

[🐚 THE SEASONS *first aid—page 170*]

Best Face

1. Always wear a sunscreen, whether it's built into your moisturizer or in a separate lotion. [page 62] **2.** Steer clear of untested products. They can lead to infections and adverse reactions. [page 168] **3.** See a dermatologist annually, especially if your skin has been damaged by the sun. Melanoma is the most easily cured cancer if it's caught early, but it can kill you if it goes untreated. [page 63] **4.** Use a night cream that is heavier than your day moisturizer. [page 58] **5.** Exfoliate at least once a week to rid skin of dead cells. [page 50] **6.** Keep hydrated. Try to drink at least eight 8-ounce glasses of noncaffeinated liquid a day. [page 29] **7.** Pay attention to your skin. If it is tight or shines, change your skin-care and makeup products. [page 50] **8.** Get a professional, deep-cleaning facial twice a year (when the seasons change). [page 170]

1. Sitting out in the sun during peak UV hours (10 a.m. to 4 p.m.). Not keeping yourself protected when you sweat and swim. [page 63] **2.** Smoking. It deprives your skin of oxygen [page 30] and causes pucker wrinkles around your lips. **3.** Using potent over-the-counter products. Try them out on a patch of skin for several days before slathering them on your face, and watch out for allergic reactions. **4.** Ignoring moles and other changes in your skin. If you're at all uncertain about anything—a rash, a patch of discoloration—see a doctor. **5.** Not protecting your skin from extreme temperature changes and cold and wind. [page 60] Wear sunglasses and a scarf. **6.** Squeezing pimples. [page 173] It's tempting, but can result in scarring and discoloration. **7.** Squinting in the sun. It's a major cause of wrinkles. Wear sunglasses. [page 60] **8.** Touching your face with dirty hands. Resting your chin, cheek, or forehead on your hands. Resting the phone against your cheek. [page 173] **9.** Not cleaning your skin every night, or overscrubbing it. Both will lead to skin problems, like breakouts. [page 50]

Worst Face

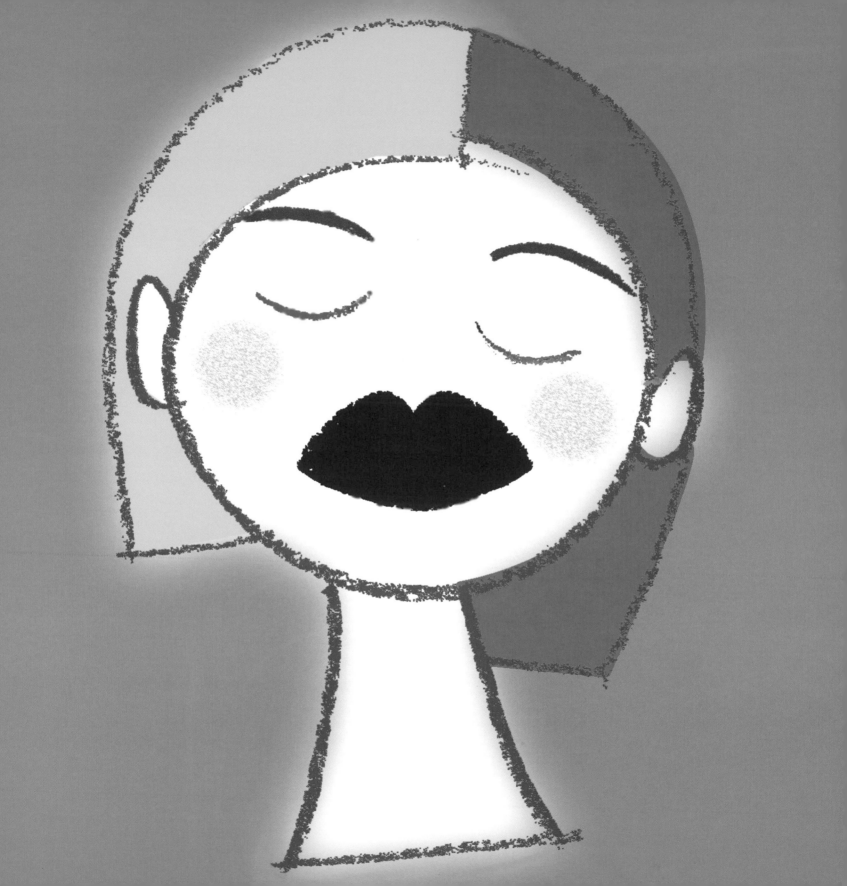

CHAPTER 4

Styling Your Makeup

How can I wear makeup without looking too made-up? [page 91] How can I update my look? [page 75] How can I create different makeup moods? [page 78] What's the easiest way to change your makeup look? [page 80] How do I create the "natural look"? [page 91] Is there a simple makeup wardrobe for everyone? [page 93] How can I dress up my day makeup for evening? [page 96]

"I love makeup. Particularly cakey, heavy, photo makeup. The get-out-the-silly-Putty-buddy-and-make-me-into-a-grown-woman-with-out-a-single-expression-line-on-my-face kind of makeup."

CLAUDIA SHEAR, *Blown Sideways Through Life*

YOUR MAKEUP PERSONALITY

Do we need makeup? In a word, no. It is not oxygen. Some of us choose to wear it to enhance our best features, a task that may be as simple as curling our eyelashes. Others may use it to help camouflage minor skin discoloration or blemishes. Still others simply have fun playing with makeup—the experimentation, the transformation. But first things first. We need to know who we are. Tomboy or glamour queen? Executive? Mother? A combination? Then we need to understand the way texture and color work to achieve different effects. Knowing what we want our look to be will help us send the message we want to send, whether it's a whisper or a shout.

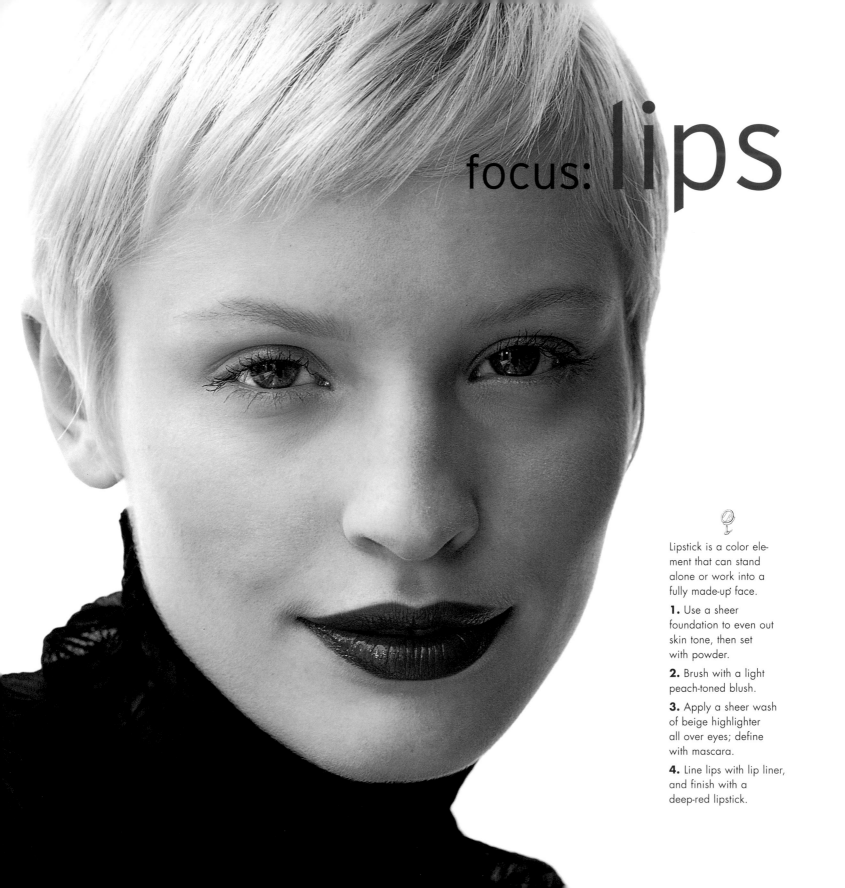

focus: lips

Lipstick is a color element that can stand alone or work into a fully made-up face.

1. Use a sheer foundation to even out skin tone, then set with powder.

2. Brush with a light peach-toned blush.

3. Apply a sheer wash of beige highlighter all over eyes; define with mascara.

4. Line lips with lip liner, and finish with a deep-red lipstick.

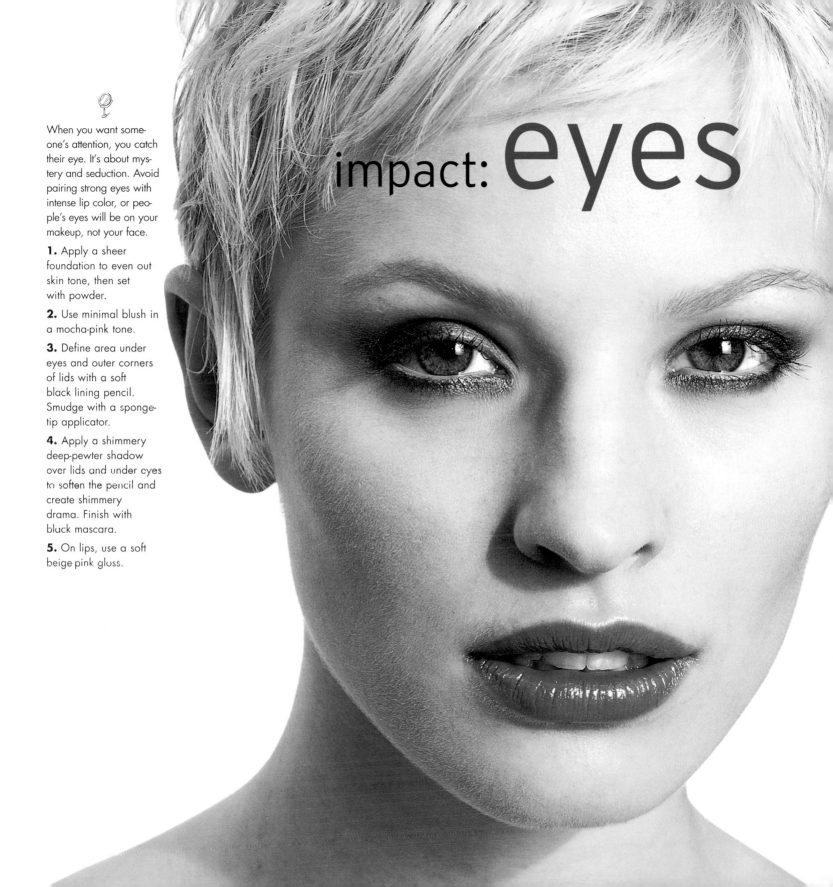

impact: eyes

When you want someone's attention, you catch their eye. It's about mystery and seduction. Avoid pairing strong eyes with intense lip color, or people's eyes will be on your makeup, not your face.

1. Apply a sheer foundation to even out skin tone, then set with powder.

2. Use minimal blush in a mocha-pink tone.

3. Define area under eyes and outer corners of lids with a soft black lining pencil. Smudge with a sponge-tip applicator.

4. Apply a shimmery deep-pewter shadow over lids and under eyes to soften the pencil and create shimmery drama. Finish with black mascara.

5. On lips, use a soft beige-pink gloss.

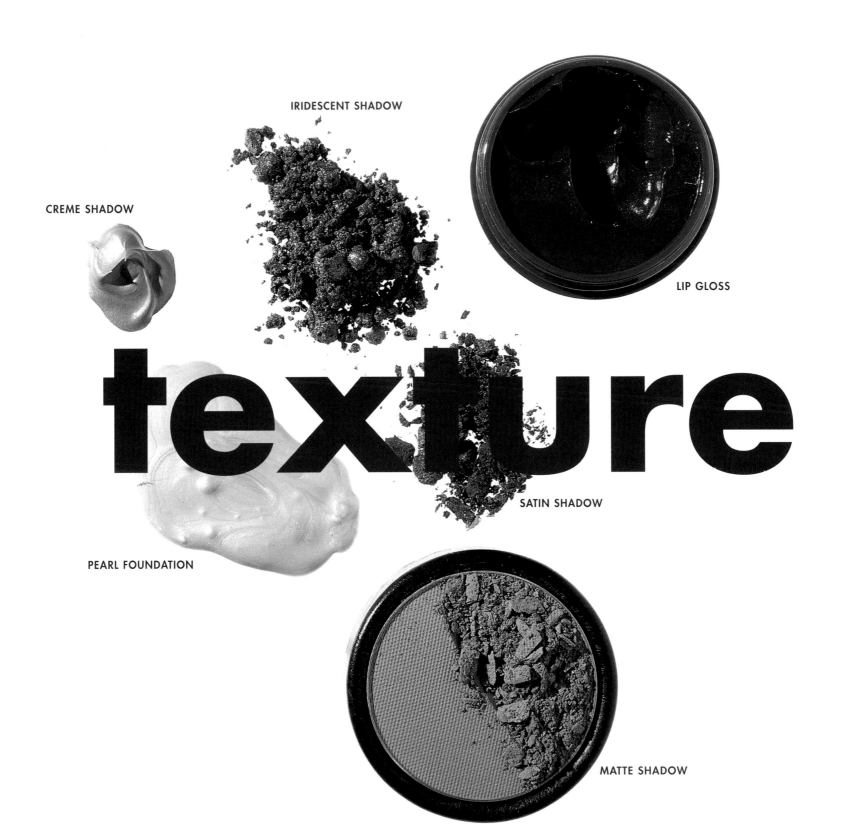

CREME SHADOW

IRIDESCENT SHADOW

LIP GLOSS

texture

PEARL FOUNDATION

SATIN SHADOW

MATTE SHADOW

A MAKEUP WARDROBE IS NOT LIKE A CLOTHING WARDROBE, WHICH IS BUILT UP OVER TIME. MAKEUP NOT ONLY GETS OLD FAST, BUT TECHNOLOGY CHANGES OUR OPTIONS FASTER THAN MANY OF US CHANGE OUR LIP color. Understanding texture will help us attain the look we desire. It's mostly about finish. Shiny. Matte. Iridescent. Sheer. It's that simple, and that complex. The same color can look completely different when you vary the texture. It can be the key to updating your look and keeping your makeup current.

MATTE is used to describe lipstick, eyeshadow, foundation, powder, and blush. It basically looks flat, with no shine whatsoever. Matte lipsticks tend to be drier but last longer. Matte foundations complement oily skin that has a shine. **SHIMMER** is the opposite of matte. It is about shine and sparkle, because shimmer cosmetics contain tiny iridescent particles. Dark skin can look superb with a slight shimmer. **SATIN** products are not as flat as matte and not as shiny as shimmer. Satin's soft, silky finish is often used to describe foundation and liquid cosmetics for the skin. Satin eyeshadows are particularly good for older skin, because they glide on smoothly **PEARLESCENT** products have some shine, yet are softer than shimmer ones. Their pearly tone can be found in eyeshadow and colorless foundation, and livens up the skin. These look especially good on Asian skin, but can look too light on dark skin. **GLOSS** is high-shine lipstick with short staying power. **IRIDESCENT** usually describes eyeshadow. It's about maximum shine and sparkle. These work best on young skin for a fun, sexy look, but can be overkill on older skins. **METALLIC** lipstick, eyeshadow, and eye pencil have a shiny metal finish. It's a downtown look that looks great on black skin but harsh on lighter and older skin. **DEWY** often refers to a foundation finish that creates a fresh and glowing look. It's great on most skins, but avoid it if you have an oily or blemished complexion. **LUMINOUS** usually describes a foundation with light-reflecting qualities that create a glowing, refined look. Luminous foundations can have a matte, satin, or dewy finish. If you have oily or blemished skin, choose matte. **SHEER** is thinner and more transparent. It can help older skin look brighter and less lined.

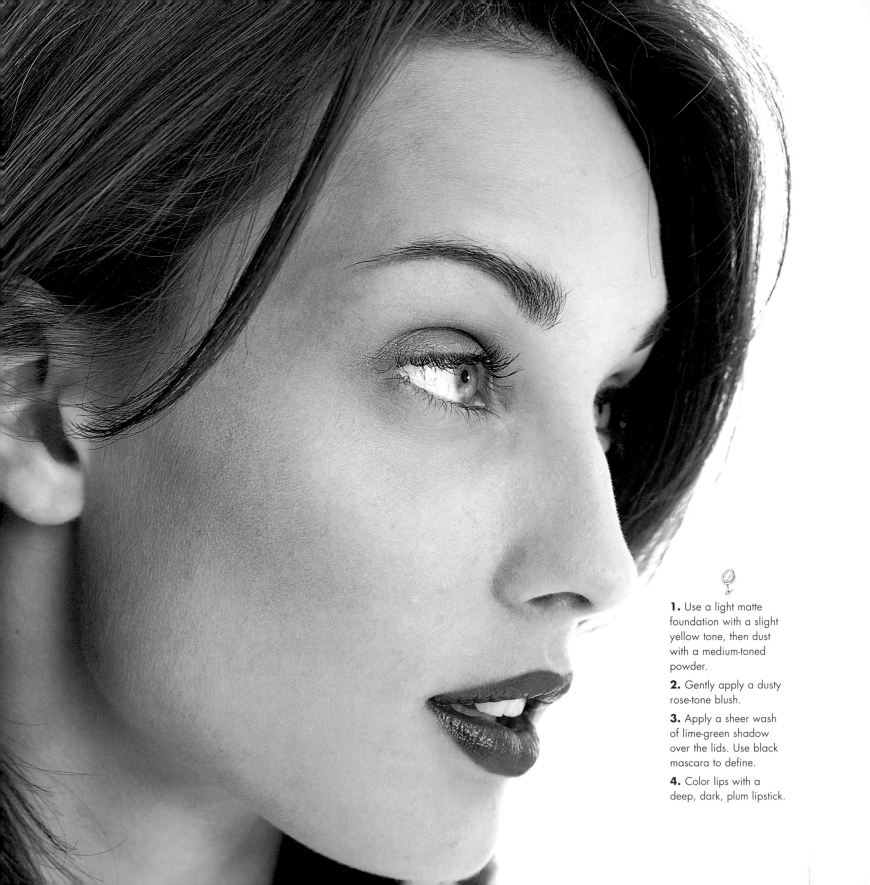

1. Use a light matte foundation with a slight yellow tone, then dust with a medium-toned powder.

2. Gently apply a dusty rose-tone blush.

3. Apply a sheer wash of lime-green shadow over the lids. Use black mascara to define.

4. Color lips with a deep, dark, plum lipstick.

color

WE START WITH OUR SKIN: IT MAY BE PALE OR RUDDY, DARK OR FAINTLY YELLOW. WHETHER WE'RE toning down redness with a yellow-tinted base or livening up our pallor with a little blush, the tone of our skin helps us determine what colors will look best on us. Hair color, regardless of where it came from, also affects the picture. When you go from being a brunette to being a blonde, you will have to rejigger your makeup a bit. A general rule: the darker your hair, the more intense color you can wear. Paler tones tend to work better with lighter hair. Your mood, your style, the season, and sometimes even the clothes you wear may also influence your choice in color. Heavy makeup tends to look out of place with a sweatshirt and jeans, just as wearing no makeup may make you look washed out if you're dressed up in black sequins.

HOW TO **WEARING COLOR ON THE EYES.** If color on your eyes brings back memories of disco queens, think again. With textures constantly evolving, today's eyeshadows are finer and more transparent, making blues, greens, and purples more wearable than ever. The key to making it work is using only one color on the eyes—leave multicolor contouring to old episodes of *Charlie's Angels.* Sweeping color over the lids with a fluffy eyeshadow brush will create a sheer wash of color. Finish with black or brown mascara to define the eye and give it more depth. The only additional color that may be needed is a soft hint of blush on the cheeks and soft, light color on the lips. Avoid strong lip color or your look will be pretty intense. If you're still nervous about color but feel like a change, look for sheer pastel or icy-pale colors. They flatter most skins and are subtle.

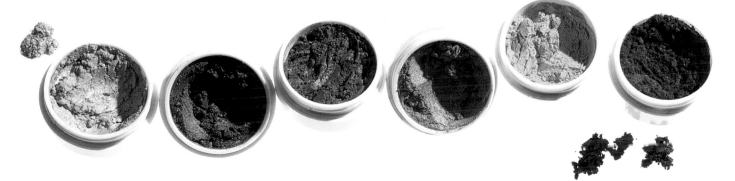

The Mix

MIXING TEXTURES BY LAYERING GIVES MAKEUP DEPTH: A METALLIC EYELINER WITH A MATTE SHADOW, OR A SPARKLING BLUSH OVER A LUMINOUS POWDER, FOR INSTANCE. TEXTURE CAN CREATE A SPECIFIC AURA: DEWY SUGGESTS YOUTHFUL; MATTE EXPRESSES SOPHISTICATION; SHIMMERY LOOKS SEXY.

HOW TO **Mixing textures and layering.** TO ACHIEVE A LUMINOUS, GLOWING EFFECT AND YOUNGER-LOOKING SKIN, mix shimmery highlighting liquid with foundation on the back of your hand with a brush. Apply as you would regular foundation. TO CREATE A CREAMY, SILKY EYESHADOW TEXTURE THAT'S EASY TO BLEND, layer matte eyeshadow over iridescent shadow. TO REVIVE OLD MATTE LIP COLORS AND MAKE THEM A LITTLE GLOSSIER, apply lip balm to your lips, then a matte lipstick. This also counters the drying effect of some matte lipsticks. TO LEND A FRESH, DEWY APPEARANCE TO OLDER SKIN, first apply tinted moisturizer all over your face, then dab creme blush on your cheeks and blend. You can also mix tinted moisturizer and creme blush together on the back of your hand, then apply the mixture to your cheeks. The result is a softer, more translucent effect.

Balancing acts. Balancing color and texture is what it's all about. Pale eyes with lots of shimmer look great with deeper colors and some shine on the lips. Darker eye makeup, where color and a more matte texture have been used for dramatic definition, looks great with a slightly dressy gloss on the lips or, for a more vintage-Hollywood effect, a simple matte red. Natural eyes, with just a wash of neutral shadow and a touch of mascara, can balance strongly colored lips with matte intensity. They also work well with lightly tinted gloss for a no-makeup effect.

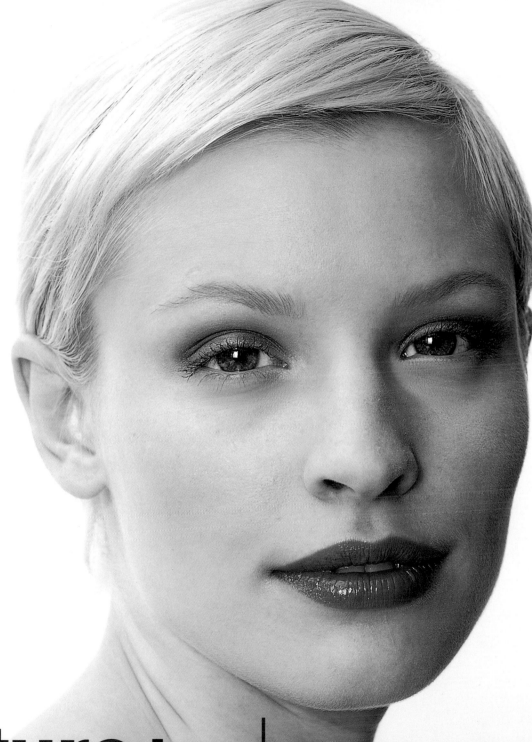

1. Brush a deep iridescent blue shadow over the lids for a vibrant wash of color.

2. Lightly apply a hint of pink powder blush.

3. Use a glossy, rose-toned lipstick.

texture+color=mood

> "You can't disguise great beauty but you can do all sorts of things with my very plain run-of-the-mill face."
>
> EMMA THOMPSON

lip color

THREE WORDS WE LIKE? QUICK. EASY. CHEAP. THAT'S THE ESSENCE OF LIP COLOR. IT'S THE QUICKEST, EASIEST, CHEAPEST WAY TO MAKE AN IMPRESSION WITH YOUR MAKEUP. IT'S ALSO A GREAT PLACE TO START

updating your makeup or experimenting with a new look. Subtle color may be perfect for mellow weekends, but for a night on the town a great red screams "Party!" Quiet, pretty shades of pink in sheer textures work well for the warmer months. In winter, we may prefer something moist and creamy in a dark-wine

Lipstick does not have to be expensive, but the price of a bad color call or two can add up. You can usually sample more expensive brands. Cheaper colors are often prepackaged, so you can't.

tone. Remember that the same shade can say very different things when you vary its texture. **Same color, new effect.** If you find a color you love, try buying it in different textures. It may look much dressier in matte than it does in sheer gloss. Alternatively, buy a matte lipstick in a color you love, then use clear lip gloss to sheer it up.

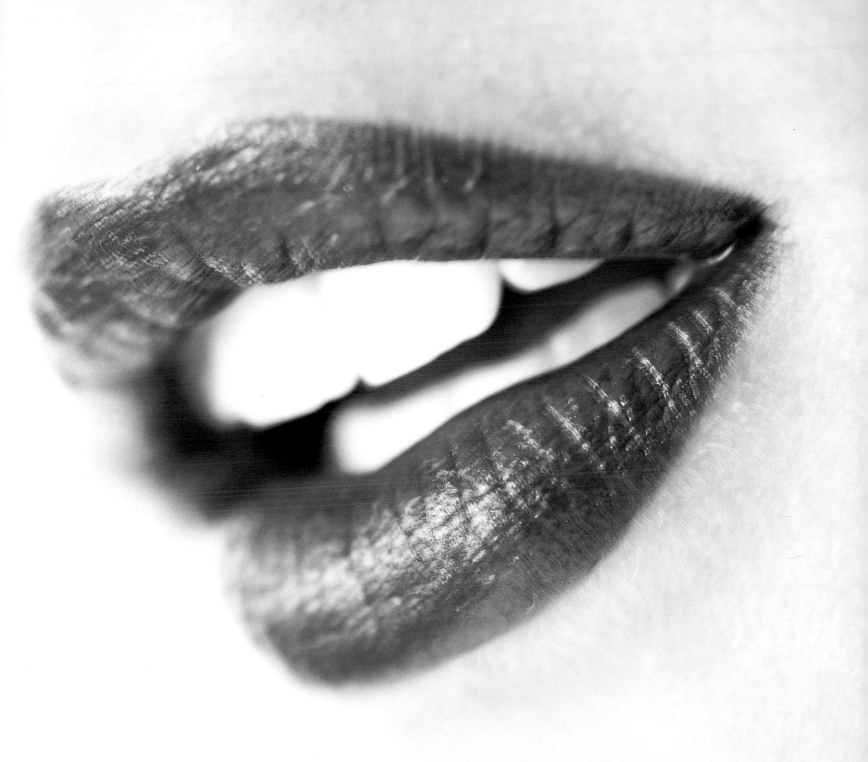

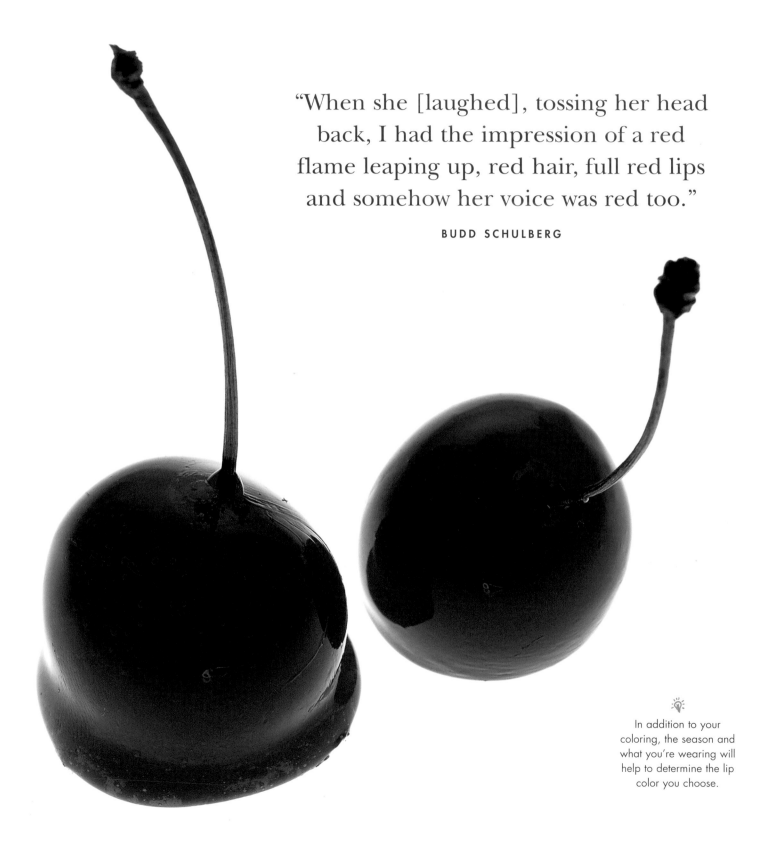

"When she [laughed], tossing her head back, I had the impression of a red flame leaping up, red hair, full red lips and somehow her voice was red too."

BUDD SCHULBERG

In addition to your coloring, the season and what you're wearing will help to determine the lip color you choose.

red

FLAPPERS IN THE 1920S GAVE PLAIN OLD RED SOME SERIOUS
ATTITUDE WHEN THEY PAINTED THEIR LIPS A DEEP CRIMSON AND ROUGED
THEIR CHEEKS, CHINS, AND EVEN THEIR EARS. RED SIGNALS A MOOD: SEXY. GLAMOROUS.

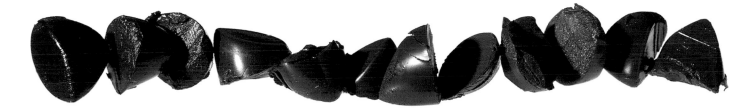

Daring. Red has become more than the hallmark of a 1950s screen siren. These days, it comes in a huge spectrum of shades. Old-fashioned deep red. Brownish mahogany. Plum. Berry. The textures of reds range from intense matte to luscious creme to the sheerest gloss. When it's deep or bright, red becomes a statement—and it's one you're likely to have strong feelings about. Maybe you hate the idea of drawing that kind of attention. Or maybe you like the appeal of wearing it with very little other makeup for a simple, modern style. It looks fresh and unexpected when worn with a white shirt and jeans. And it says instant evening with a black cocktail dress.

Strong reds can look severe and aging on **MATURE FACES.** Look for muted shades in a creamy texture that won't dry out your lips. Soft berry reds with a bluish undertone go with **FAIR SKIN.** Deeper plum reds can also look great. Stay away from orange tones, as they can appear aging. **REDHEADS** look beautiful in soft brownish reds, apricot, and sheer raisin shades. Richer, deeper reds are flattering to **MEDIUM SKIN.** For yellow undertones, blue reds will brighten and brown reds will look warmer. **OLIVE** or **YELLOW-TONED SKIN** looks terrible in pink or orange reds. Stick with deep brownish reds or dark berry tones. **BLACK SKIN** looks best with deep blue-toned and mahogany reds. Avoid pink and orange reds.

pink

REMINISCENT OF BUBBLE GUM AND COTTON CANDY, PINK WAS PROBABLY THE COLOR OF YOUR FIRST lipstick. Soft enough to be innocent, but sweet enough to inspire that first kiss (and subsequent blush). Pink should be about looking pretty, but there's a danger to wearing the color of your youth. Frosted opaques, vivid fuchsias, and candy-colored shades may work on young faces, but on more mature women they can look dated and drain color from your skin. Muted pinks in warmer tones flatter almost any skin tone. Pink is a fleeting, seasonal color, though. Once the flowers stop blooming, it's time to move on to more subdued shades—at least until next spring.

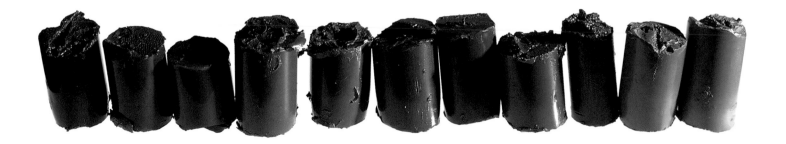

Light, transparent pinks look best on **FAIR SKIN.** They can be pale and glossy, with a slight blue undertone, or muted and dusty, with a subtle hint of beige. **REDHEADS** usually have delicate red undertones, making most pinks hard to wear. The exceptions are peachy and apricot pinks, salmon, and sheer red-pink glosses. **MEDIUM SKIN** looks best with deeper, warmer pinks that have soft mauve, blue, or brown undertones. **OLIVE** and **YELLOW-TONED SKINS** have strong yellow undertones, so avoid light pinks, as they can look draining. Deep rose, berry, and soft plum pinks look best. Strong pinks don't work with **BLACK SKIN.** Instead, go for soft, sheer, nude pinks. Glossy beiges with a hint of pink can look wonderful on dark skin. Lighter black skin usually has golden undertones, and colors that are too pale should be avoided. Deep rose, berry, and plum tones look best.

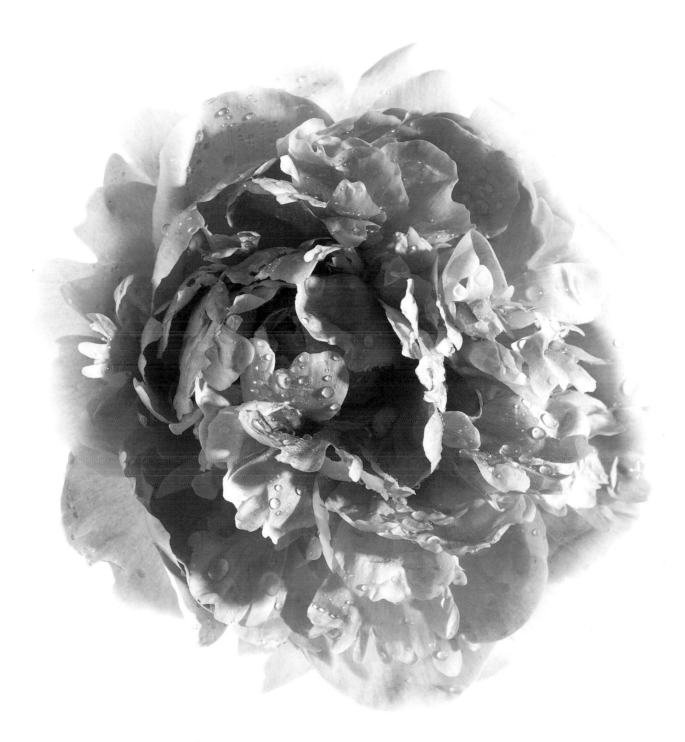

☀ Pink foundation and powders will make your skin look older.

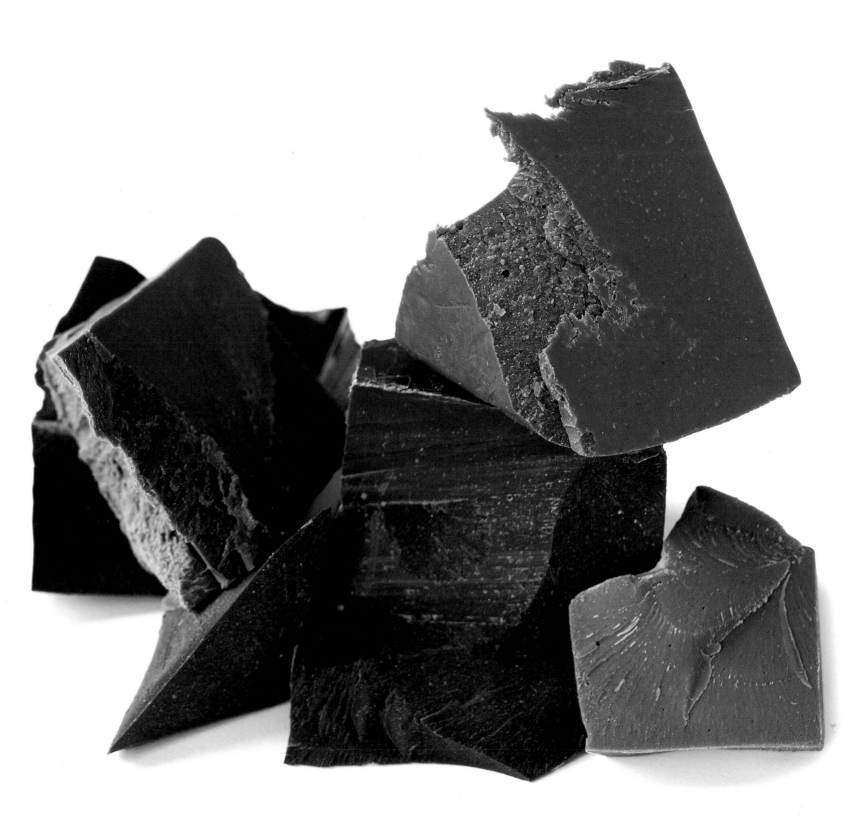

Brown

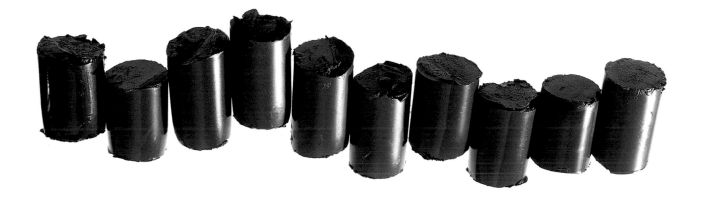

BEFORE THE 1980S, CHOCOLATE WAS SOMETHING YOU PUT IN YOUR MOUTH, NOT ON YOUR LIPS. BUT THEN, IN THE AFTERMATH OF DISCO GLITTER, EARTH TONES RULED, AND BROWN CAME INTO ITS OWN. IT'S TAKEN A WHILE TO perfect the shades and textures. It began as a dark, muddy sludge tone, one that made you look either half-dead or as if you'd been eating dirt. No longer. Natural and subtly glamorous, the new browns range from rich coffee to pale beige. Textures that are sheerer allow for some natural lip color to come through, resulting in a softer, livelier look. The result? A good brown will take you from business meeting to cocktail party to weekend supper. Subtle and flexible, it is becoming a makeup-wardrobe basic.

On **FAIR SKIN,** pink-toned beiges, honey shades, and mocha browns work well. Deeper chocolate browns create drama for stronger evening looks. **REDHEADS** should stick with sheer raisin or peachy hues. For more dramatic color, try rich browns with red undertones. Beiges and pink browns can clash with pale skin and red hair. **MEDIUM SKIN** can look washed out with browns that are too pale and beige. Soft mocha, coffee, and caramel colors work best. For **OLIVE** and **YELLOW-TONED SKIN,** varying shades of chocolate, toffee, and mahogany, and browns with red or plum undertones offer depth and sexy drama. **BLACK SKIN** was made to wear brown, from the ultralight, glossy beiges to the deepest chocolate.

wearing browns

Overall effect:
sophisticated, modern everyday glamour

1. On the cheeks, a soft, honey-toned blush for a hint
of warmth and shape (blush: see page 120).

2. Dark-brown pencil/shadow liner used
to give depth and definition to the eye
(eye pencil: see page 128).

3. Shimmery, chocolate-bronze shadow applied on lids and
under eyes to soften the pencil and give a smudgy,
shimmery look (eyeshadow: see page 131).

4. Strong, glossy lips in a rich cinnamon.
The gloss helps soften the color's impact (lips: see page 136).

What if I want to experiment with fashion makeup colors?
Generally, the younger you are, the more trends you can wear. If you're older, trendy colors may call
attention to your age unless you wear them simply and minimally in sheer or subtle textures. Be selective
about where you apply them. For example, a color with a purple tone is easier to wear on the lips than the
eyes, while a shimmery gold highlighter on the eyes works for most skin tones.

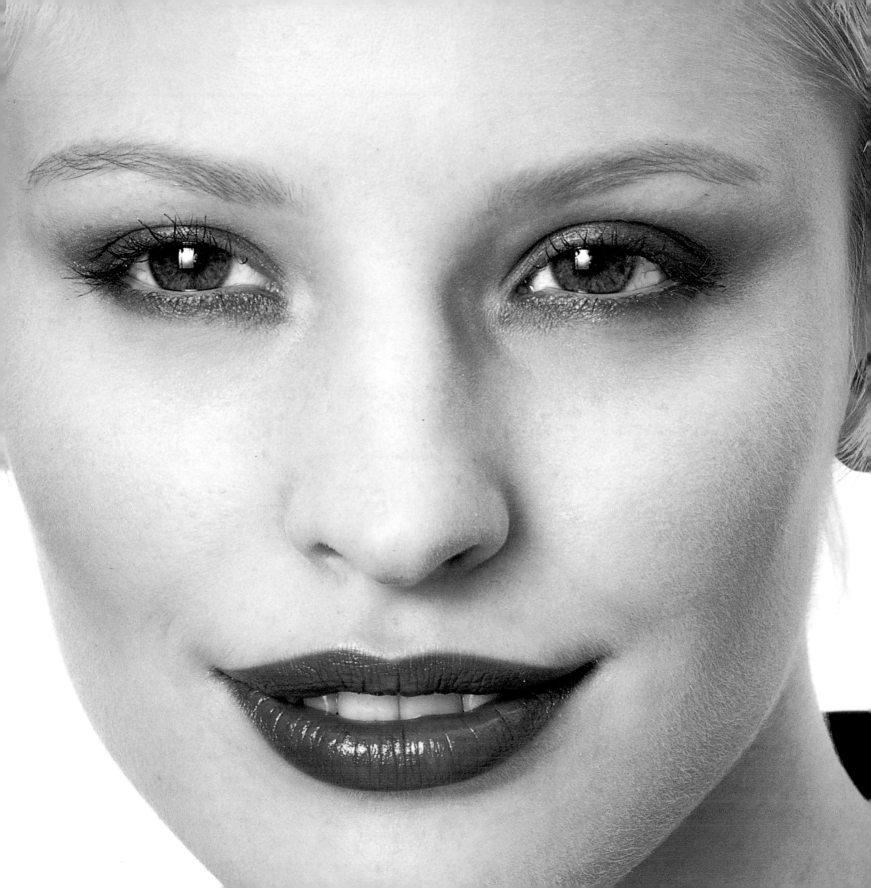

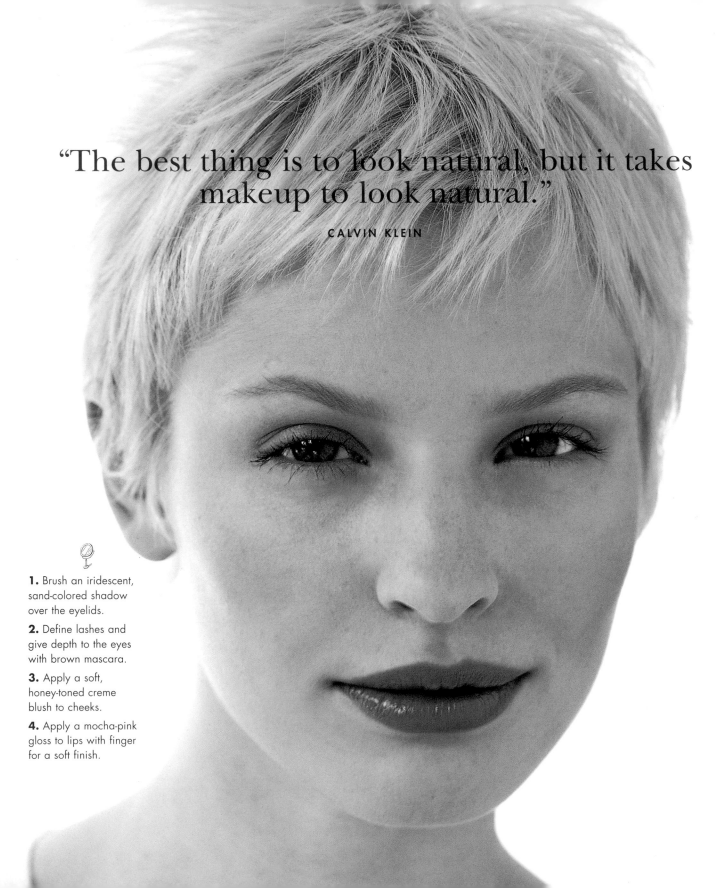

"The best thing is to look natural, but it takes makeup to look natural."

CALVIN KLEIN

1. Brush an iridescent, sand-colored shadow over the eyelids.

2. Define lashes and give depth to the eyes with brown mascara.

3. Apply a soft, honey-toned creme blush to cheeks.

4. Apply a mocha-pink gloss to lips with finger for a soft finish.

natural

NATURAL-LOOKING MAKEUP IS DESIGNED TO ENHANCE WHAT MOTHER NATURE GAVE you without making a makeup "statement." It's not just about the amount of makeup you may choose to wear. It's more about using subtle colors that are highly transparent, so your skin color will glow through, rather than appearing washed out. **COLOR.** This is not about bright colors or dark colors. It's about shades in subtle tones of mocha, sand, peach, and pinkish-beige.

TEXTURE. Stay away from flat opaques. Textures to use are transparent, glossy, sheer, and slightly iridescent. Because of their transparency, the same shades will look different on each person's skin. On **FAIR SKIN**, naturals should look warm and pale. The radiance of **BLACK SKIN** can be enhanced with a soft, pale iridescence. **OLIVE** and **YELLOW-TONED** skin demand a deeper-brown lip color, with some sheen for soft, glossy definition. But generally, natural colors work for all skins if they're transparent and sheer and allow your natural coloring to come through.

Universal Makeup

Sheer texture + Neutral color

DARK OLIVE SKIN

Eyeshadow applied with a sponge tip for more concentrated definition. Balm applied over lipstick for a glossy finish.

REDHEAD

Eyeshadow applied with a fluffy brush for a sheer wash of color. Lip color diluted with balm. Very soft blush on cheeks.

BRUNETTE

Lipstick applied directly emphasizes the lips. A sheer wash of silvery taupe eyeshadow is brushed on.

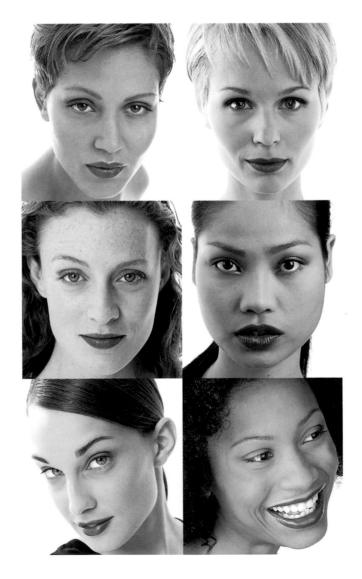

BLONDE

Dark-brown pencil defines the eyes. Eyeshadow applied over pencil softens the effect, and adds depth.

ASIAN

Eyeshadow applied all over lid with a sponge tip and under the eye with an eyeliner brush for increased definition. Lipstick applied with a brush for a sheerer texture.

BLACK

Layers of blush give more tone. Dark-brown pencil at base of eye at outer corners gives definition. Eyeshadow applied with sponge tip for a soft but defined eye. Lipstick applied with a brush, blotted, then reapplied for purer color.

ONE MAKEUP WARDROBE THAT WORKS FOR EVERYONE. EVERY AGE, EVERY COLOR. NO-BRAINER MAKEUP. THE COLORS ARE NEUTRALS, BASED ON BROWNS. THE TEXTURES HAVE A DELICATE VIBRANCY, AND AREN'T DULL OR FLAT. IT is makeup with a soft sheen and a texture that is almost transparent. It enlivens the skin while allowing its natural color to come through, so it looks different on each person. What makes these colors work on everyone has to do with how you put them on. They can be worn subtly, or layered for more definition drama. By having the right tools and practicing, you can achieve different looks with the same colors.

HOW TO **BLUSH.** A fine, sheer powder in a warm, rosy brown will give a soft whisper of color. On darker skins, layer color gradually for more tone. **EYESHADOW.** Deep copper-brown and silver-brownish taupe eyeshadows are rich and silky. A hint of shine makes them easier to blend. A subtle, creamy banana-colored highlighter can work in several places: on the brow bone, on lids, or layered with another shadow (the lighter one first) for a lighter effect. For a sheer wash of color over the eyelid, use a fluffy eyeshadow brush. A sponge-tip applicator gives more definition. Deep copper-brown shadow is rich and gives depth; silver-brown taupe is softer, sheerer, and lends a subtle tone. Both work with all eye colors. **EYE PENCIL.** A soft, powdery dark brown, it emphasizes eyes, creates depth, and can look like eyeshadow when well blended. **LIPS.** Lip colors are in deep tones of brownish red, brownish pink, and plum brown. The textures are sheer and glossy. If they're applied straight from the lipstick, the color will be denser. Mixing your lip color with lip balm can create a sheerer texture.

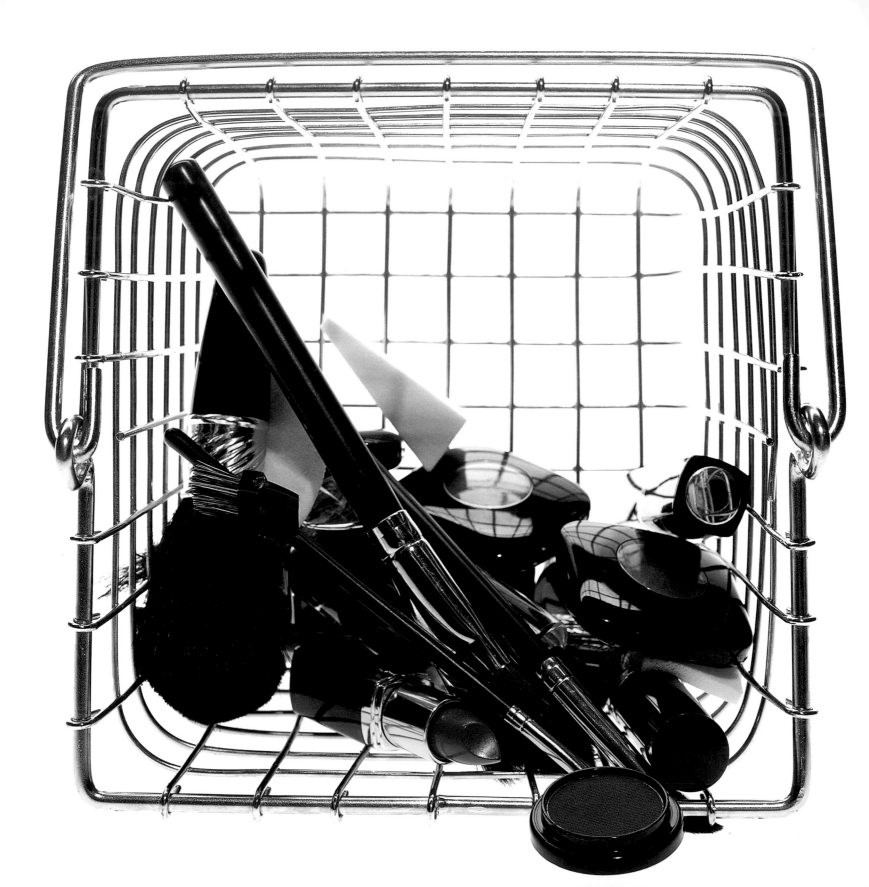

How **much money** should you spend?

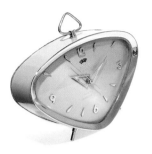

Are You Stuck in Time?

YOU ARE DRESSING YOUR FACE. YOU ARE SLATHERING ON CLEANSERS, TONERS, AND MOISTURIZERS. OCCASIONALLY, YOU MIGHT FIND yourself embalmed in a seaweed mask. You rub in colored creams you hope will make you look radiant, dewy, velvety—you name your texture. You are dusting your pores with powder and brushing a dark paste over your lashes. Since this is all going onto your skin, it's worth going out of your way to find exactly the right products that work for you and make you look the way you dream of looking. Your basic makeup wardrobe is what you depend on, day in, day out. There are some items you can't skimp on—foundation, for one: it's crucial that you get a high-quality foundation that exactly matches your skin tone. But the mascaras, eyeliners, and lip liners you can find at a drugstore usually do the job just as capably as the more expensive versions found at department store cosmetic counters.

Sometimes we cling to the past. We've been there, it's familiar, and we know we once looked great in liquid eyeliner or frosted lipstick…didn't we? Sticking with makeup simply because it's what you've worn since your high school prom is not a good idea. Each age should be a celebration of who you are today, not a memorial to who you were back then. Your face, your hair, your body—they're all different now, and you need to adjust the way you care for them, as well as the way you enhance them. But you're not the only one who's evolved. Makeup has, too. The homespun potions of antiquity have paved the way for foundations that protect us from the sun, mascaras that condition and lengthen our lashes, and lipsticks that moisturize while adding color. Makeup today should be less of a mask and more of a second skin. It considers our sensitivities, our breakouts, our contact lenses, and our age. It can be confusing, but there's a better chance of finding the perfect makeup now than ever before. And if that means we don't have to go around looking like we just fell out of a time capsule, who's complaining?

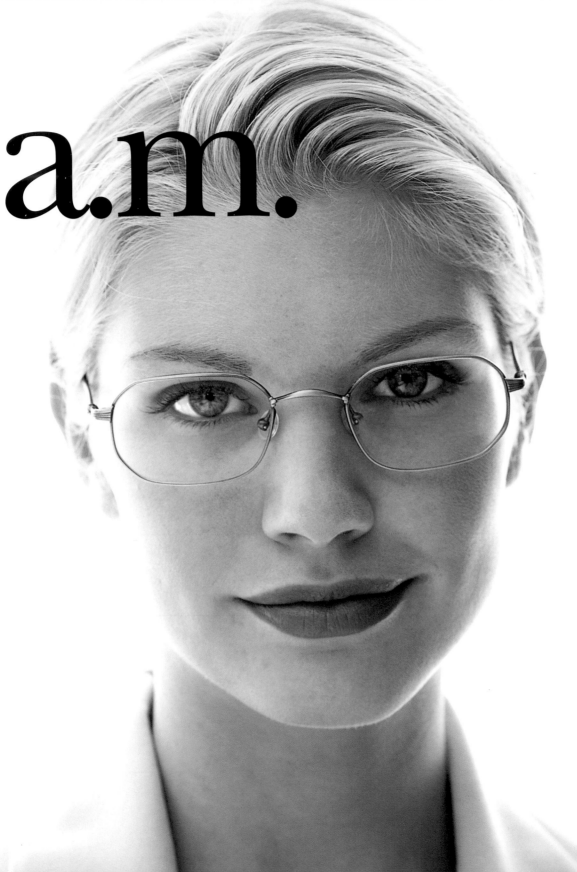

a.m.

TRANSFORMATION

1. Spray your face with water. Wipe off surface powder and dull-looking makeup with a cotton pad.

2. Use a wide, flat foundation brush to apply foundation where needed. Blend lightly with a dry latex wedge.

3. Brush on loose powder all over.

4. Apply blush to the apples of your cheeks.

5. Use a latex wedge to clean up eye makeup and press loose powder in the area around eyes and nose.

6. Define the outer corners of the lid at the base of the lashes using a soft lining pencil. Fade out edges and smudge the pencil line inward with a sponge-tip applicator.

7. Apply a neutral, shimmery shadow over the pencil.

8. Recurl lashes.

9. Add a coat of mascara.

10. Apply lip color and top with gloss for evening shine.

FROM WORK TO PLAY
Part of choosing what kind of makeup to wear will depend on where you are going. Your choices may vary according to whether you're off to the office, your kids' soccer match, or a wedding. You might start with very little in the morning, then add on a layer in the evening.

"She had two complexions, A.M. and P.M."

RING LARDNER

p.m.

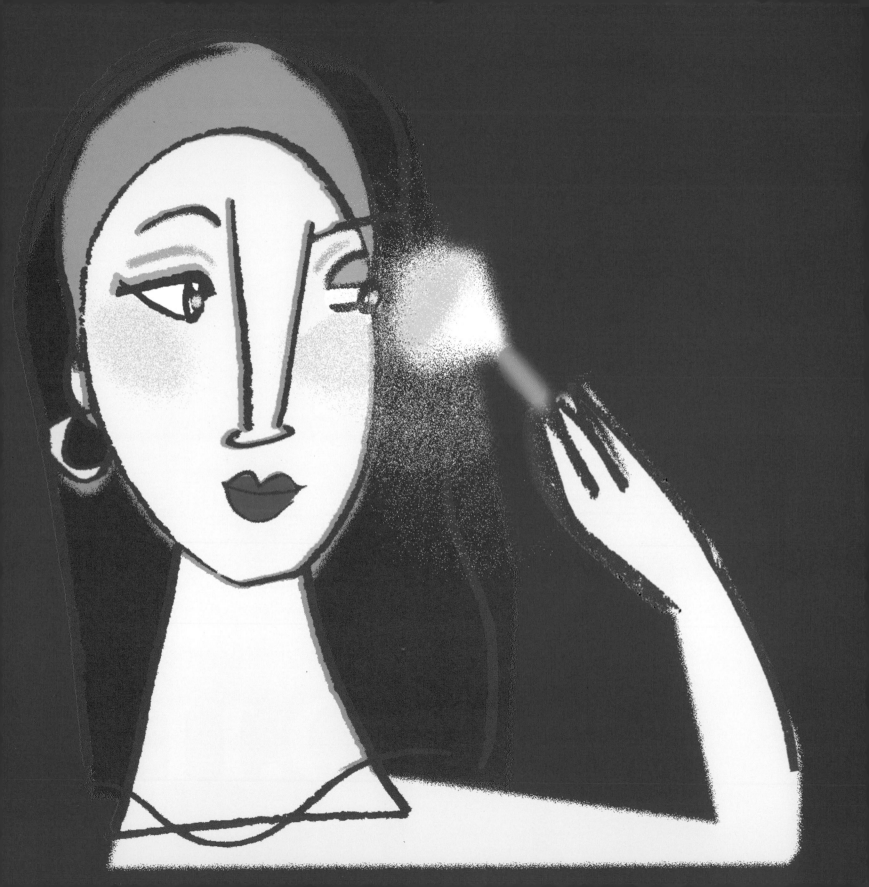

Putting On Your Makeup

"I HAVE FOUND IN THE PAST THAT IF YOU BUM RUSH THE TRANSFORMATION, YOU GET LESS THAN STELLAR RESULTS. BREATHING, RELAXING, BEING CALM— THIS IS HALF OF WHAT IT'S ALL ABOUT. THE TRANSFORMATION IS BOTH PHYSICAL AND MENTAL. THE GODDESS IS AS MUCH A STATE OF MIND AS A LOOK."

RuPAUL, *Lettin' It All Hang Out*

SIMPLE TECHNIQUES

Okay, you've done enough evaluating. Now it's time for action. Simplicity is everything. Minimal tools. Easy application. The exact products you need, nothing more. In this chapter, we go over the nuts and bolts of putting on your makeup. What is the difference between a powder brush and a blush brush? How do you get your makeup to stay on throughout the day? How can you minimize under-eye circles? The idea is to get your makeup routine down to the point where it is fast and easy—almost automatic. That process begins here.

1 FOUNDATION. As the base that evens out your complexion and covers small irregularities, your foundation's tone depends largely on your own skin. Is your skin looking radiant and beautiful without help? Then skip the foundation and go for a light dusting of loose powder.

2 CONCEALER. A miracle paste that hides everything your foundation didn't—from broken capillaries and under-eye circles to telltale signs of an occasional chocolate binge. No trouble spots? No need. **3 POWDER.** For setting foundation, giving your face a smooth finish, and keeping shine under control, powder is indispensable. It is not a step to skip. You can even brush it over a clean, moisturized face for a fresh, no-makeup look. Makeup won't last the day without powder. **4 BLUSH.** For adding a warm glow and a little shaping to your face. If your cheeks are naturally rosy, then you may choose to leave things to Mother Nature and skip the blush.

5 BROWS. Shaped and groomed to define your eyes, they project mood and expression. Don't overlook this step, as it is important in determining your overall look. **6 EYELINER.** For defining and bringing out your eyes. **7 EYESHADOW.** A light wash of color, or a more dramatic layering of color and texture to define your eyes. **8 MASCARA.** To give you the lashes you wish you had: full, long, thick, and dark. Sometimes just using an eyelash curler is all it takes to spotlight your baby blues (or browns or hazels or greens).

9 LIP COLOR. It's the quickest way to add a little color and set the mood for your overall look. Go all out for defined lips and long-lasting color by lining them, then coloring them in. Or smear on a clear gloss or a healing lip balm for a pared-down, natural look.

[🧰 SURVIVAL GEAR *first aid—page 164*]

what makeup can do for **you**

TOOLS

MICHELANGELO DID NOT PAINT THE CEILING OF THE SISTINE CHAPEL WITH HIS FINGER. HE NEEDED TOOLS, AND SO DO YOU. BUY GOOD-QUALITY, NATURAL-HAIR BRUSHES. YOU WILL BE ABLE TO CONTROL your makeup better, it will take you less time to apply your makeup, and your makeup will stay on longer. Your home set should be full-size, but a mini-size kit is perfect if you're on the road a lot. Even expensive makeup can look streaky and overdone if it's put on with the wrong tools. Invest in a few choice brushes, and no one will ever think you used a trowel.

A SHARPENER just like the one in your old school pencil case, only this one's for lip and eye pencils. Pop soft pencils in the freezer for a few minutes before sharpening to prevent them from breaking in the sharpener. A note of caution: a sharpener made by one cosmetic company may not work with the eye pencil of another. You need **TWEEZERS** for cleaning up brows. Look for a pair you can hold easily, with scissor handles or a finger grip. Avoid pointed tips, which can pinch your skin. **A BROW BRUSH** helps to tame brow hairs and soften brow makeup. Armed with an **EYELASH CURLER** and a steady hand, you can crimp lashes upward to make them look longer. Place curler at base of lashes, and be careful not to pull or break hairs. Do not curl for longer than 15 seconds. Apply mascara after curling, and wash the rubber curling pad often. **COTTON SWABS** are perfect for blending and for removing mascara mistakes. **TISSUES** are excellent for cleaning brushes and for wiping up spills, but use them sparingly to blot skin—the wood fiber they are made from can irritate sensitive skin. **LATEX WEDGES** are perfect for cleaning up smudges under the eyes and powdering the eyelids to help eyeshadow last longer. Use it like an eraser to tone down heavy makeup and remove smudges. Keep a couple in your daily kit to clean up old makeup and to tone down shine with powder. When damp, a small **SEA SPONGE** will help to give a soft, even finish to foundation by blending it more easily.

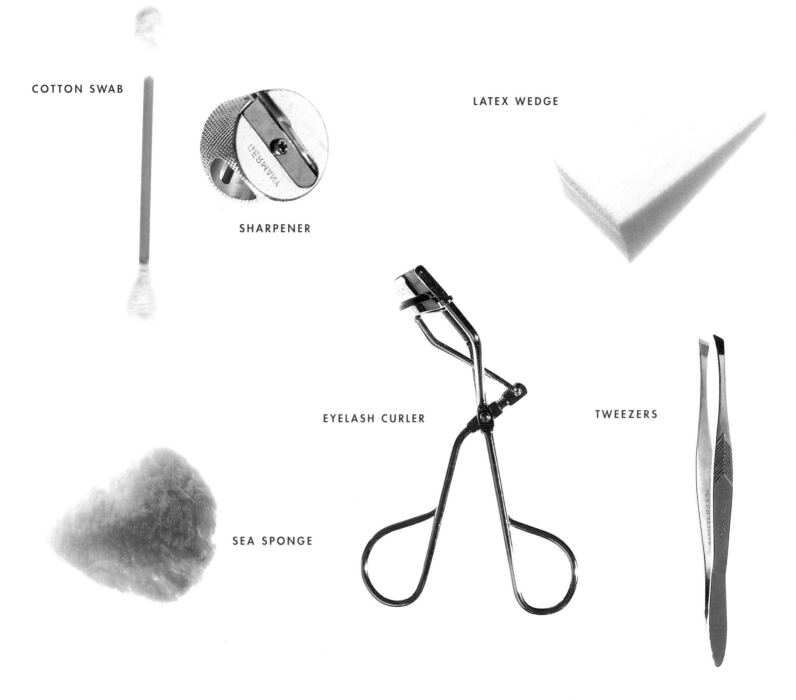

COTTON SWAB

SHARPENER

LATEX WEDGE

EYELASH CURLER

SEA SPONGE

TWEEZERS

"One of the things that gets me hot is having a Q-Tip in my ear."

ANDY WARHOL

TOOLS

EYESHADOW BRUSH
A fluffy brush that is tapered with a rounded head. Used for applying a sheer wash of shadow. Also good for blending, and for removing shadow when you've put too much on. Look for one with soft, supple hair.

SPONGE-TIP APPLICATOR
When applying eyeshadow, sponges can create more controlled definition than brushes. They also help prevent shadow from falling around the eye, and are ideal for blending eye pencil for a smooth finish.

FOUNDATION BRUSH
The flatness of a foundation brush enables you to apply a thinner layer wherever it's needed. It's also great for mixing foundation with concealer or applying concealer close to the eye.

CLEANING BRUSHES
If used daily, brushes should be cleaned once a week. Otherwise the hairs will be damaged and it will be more difficult to apply makeup. Wash gently with shampoo and warm water, being careful not to rub the hairs the wrong way. Rinse well, and smooth hairs into place, then let air-dry (larger brushes may need up to two days' drying time). Or use a makeup dry-cleaning solution by pouring it onto a tissue, then gently wiping across the brush. Brushes will dry immediately.

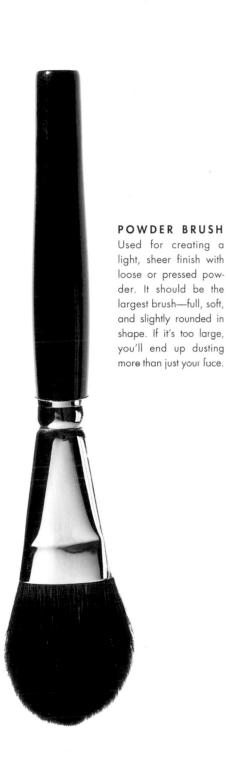

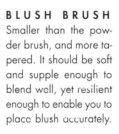

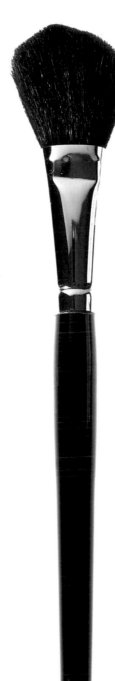

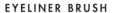

BROW BRUSH
In a pinch, a clean (preferably new) toothbrush can substitute.

POWDER BRUSH
Used for creating a light, sheer finish with loose or pressed powder. It should be the largest brush—full, soft, and slightly rounded in shape. If it's too large, you'll end up dusting more than just your face.

BLUSH BRUSH
Smaller than the powder brush, and more tapered. It should be soft and supple enough to blend well, yet resilient enough to enable you to place blush accurately.

BRUSH SELECTION
Invest in good-quality brushes, like those made from sable. They ensure better results, and, with care, they will last longer.

EYELINER BRUSH
Used to soften and blend pencil around the eye. Also good for applying eyeshadow as liner, wet or dry, and for painting concealer over blemishes.

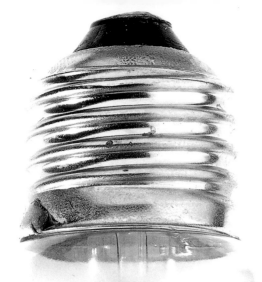

Light

"LUX ET VERITAS" — *Motto of Yale University*

UNLESS YOU WORK THE NIGHT SHIFT UNDER A STRING OF FLUORESCENT LIGHTS, YOUR MAKEUP WILL BE SEEN BY MOST PEOPLE IN NATURAL LIGHT—SO YOU SHOULD APPLY IT IN A LIGHT THAT'S AS SIMILAR to sunlight as possible. Ideally, that would mean setting up your makeup table near a large window, preferably with a pastoral view of a rolling green landscape. Unfortunately, it's probably a little outside your makeup budget to blast through the bathroom wall and install that window. Most of us have to make the best of the lighting we have, but there are interesting options: at some makeup salons and lighting stores you can find special bulbs that give off full-spectrum, close-to-natural light. They're more expensive, but they can be worth it.

CHROMALUX BULB. The closest thing to natural light this side of the sun, the Chromalux bulb blocks out yellow tones to lend a warmer, more natural glow to your skin. **IN A GOOD LIGHT.** The most flattering light hits your face at a 45-degree angle; the least flattering light comes from above or below and casts shadows around your eyes. **THE PERFECT HUE.** With colored light, light blue and amber can be flattering. Shy away from red, darker blue, green, and bright yellow.

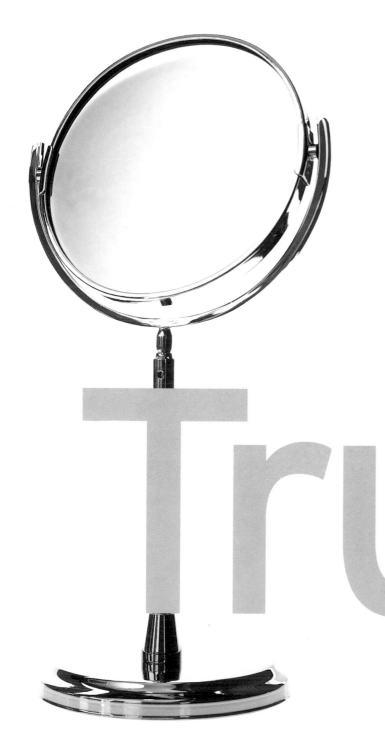

IRONICALLY, A PIECE OF YOUR COSMETIC ARSENAL THAT'S OFTEN OVERLOOKED IS RIGHT IN FRONT OF YOUR face: the mirror. It's the gauge by which you measure the effectiveness of all your other products, so it needs to be of high quality. Make sure that your mirror is thick enough, so it won't distort. The clarity of the glass and brilliance of the silvering also vary—as does the strength of the backing, which affects the mirror's durability. Magnifying mirrors can be helpful if you normally wear glasses, but they can also cause distortion and exaggerate minor imperfections, ultimately leading you to wear too much makeup. Look for models that attach to your bathroom mirror with clips or suction cups. The best mirrors can be found at good glass stores. Remember, too, not to tilt a full-length mirror against the wall. You'll think you're in a fun house.

WE ARE NOT BORN WITH THE UNCHANGING COMPLEXION OF A WAX FIGURINE. OUR FACES ARE FULL OF THE FLAWS THAT MAKE US HUMAN. BUT MAKEUP OFTEN NEEDS A BASE, A CLEAN CANVAS, WHERE SUBTLE

textures and colors on the eyes, cheeks, and lips can shine. Foundation is the key. It evens out the skin tone and can conceal small imperfections. In fact, it may be the only makeup you choose to wear, so deciding on just the right formula and color can be one of the toughest challenges you face when you're building a makeup wardrobe. Ask yourself a few questions. Is your skin tone fair, olive, or dark? Do you have dry, oily, or combination skin? Do you want the natural sheen of light coverage, or do you prefer the perfect matte finish of a *Sunset Boulevard* closeup? Do you want sun protection? How much time and money are you willing to spend to look flawless? Foundation and powder are the two components that experts agree are worth the investment. Prepackaged formulas are usually available in only a limited number of colors, and cannot be tested before buying. If you get this part wrong, it can ruin everything that follows.

Yellow-based foundations work well on everyone. No, you won't look jaundiced. In fact, if you have naturally yellow-toned skin, you should avoid foundations that are too white, or else you'll look ashen and chalky. Foundations with a little yellow will even out every complexion and blend into natural coloring. In addition, yellow minimizes red, which may be an element of your coloring as a result of tanning, broken capillaries, or aging.

FOUND

Color. It sounds easy: your base should complement your complexion. If you choose the right color, it will look as though it has disappeared into your skin. Most skin is slightly yellow-toned or ruddy, so your foundation should have yellow undertones, not pink. The same goes for pink or more reddish complexions: a yellow-based foundation helps tone down high coloring. Avoid pink or orange tones, unless you want to look like you're wearing a mask. The most natural looks have beige, neutral, or yellow undertones, and they should disappear into your natural skin color. An obvious line between your foundation and your natural skin color means that your foundation is the wrong color. Try fingerprints of several colors on the side of your face, just above the jaw. Don't rub the test streaks into your skin. Lightly fade out the edges so that you can see the true color of the base. If none of the shades work, ask about custom blending. Two things to remember: first, unless you spend most of your time under a grow-light, try to assess your options in natural daylight. Another option is natural-daylight bulbs or a soft white light. And remember that you may have to adapt your foundation shade to fit seasonal changes in your skin tone.

LIQUID FOUNDATION is the most popular formula. It's easy to use and looks natural. Apply with a foundation brush.

FOUND

Formulation. The formula of your base should complement your skin type. Oil-free foundation is good for **ALL SKIN TYPES,** especially oily complexions, or skin that breaks out easily. For very **OILY SKIN,** there are special oil-absorbent formulations available. A moisturizing base can help **DRY SKIN** that tends to flake under makeup. Tinted moisturizers, with or without an oil base, are the sheerest foundations available. Their luminous texture is ideal for **DELICATE SKIN,** which may look overdone in anything but the lightest makeup. They also work well in the summer, or for a simple light coverage.

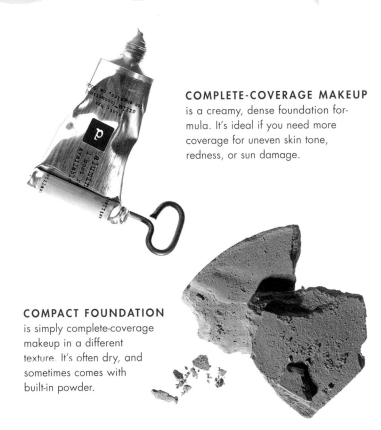

COMPLETE-COVERAGE MAKEUP is a creamy, dense foundation formula. It's ideal if you need more coverage for uneven skin tone, redness, or sun damage.

COMPACT FOUNDATION is simply complete-coverage makeup in a different texture. It's often dry, and sometimes comes with built-in powder.

LIQUID is good for all skin types. Liquid foundations come in oil-free and moisturizing formulas, with different levels of coverage depending on the brand. Generally they look the most natural. **CREME** is specially formulated for drier complexions. It is thicker, offering more coverage, but can be thinned after application by blending with a damp sponge. Creme bases tend to lie heavier on the skin than liquids and may emphasize fine lines around the eyes. For fast coverage, **COMPACT** foundation is available in two formulations. A combination creme-and-powder goes on wet as a base and dries to a powder, so you can skip the powder step. The other type is a creme formula that gives more coverage. Beware: dry skin can look cakey under these foundations, and results can be slightly flat and heavy looking. **STICK** foundation is ideal for maximum coverage of scars, birthmarks, and larger imperfections. It is essentially a creme foundation and concealer in one neat package. Sticks can speed up your application time but will look like overkill on clear skin. **TINTED MOISTURIZER** is the sheerest of them all and is especially good for summer. It offers minimum coverage, which varies from brand to brand, and it's ideal for those who don't like the feel of makeup but want a little color. **SHEER FACE TINT** usually gives a little more coverage than a tinted moisturizer, and evens out the skin tone in a subtle way. It is available in moisturizing and oil-free formulas.

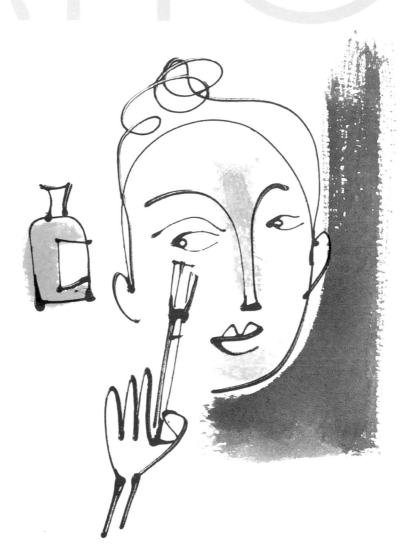

What is the shelf life of the average foundation? Most are good for about a year. After that, look for signs of clumping, darkening, and separation. Old makeup may also smell bad.

Before applying, allow your moisturizer to sink into your skin for a few minutes. **STEP 1.** For a more natural look, apply base with a foundation brush wherever it's needed, usually in the middle part of the face—cheeks, nose, forehead, chin—and on any problem areas. It's not necessary to apply it all the way to your hairline. Applying a little foundation to the inside corners of your eyes creates the illusion that your eyes are brighter. If the foundation is sheer, you may want to blend it lightly over your eyelids to even out your coloring—but bear in mind that this can make your eye makeup crease. **STEP 2.** Use a small, slightly damp sea sponge to spread the base more thinly over the skin. This will also keep oil-free foundation from drying before you blend it, and will help prevent foundation from clinging to patches of dry skin. **STEP 3.** Brush on loose powder to set foundation and prevent shine.

"Look like th' innocent flower,
But be the serpent under't."

LADY MACBETH

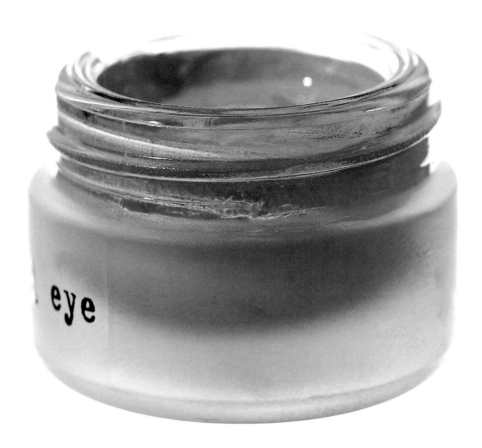

eye

SOLID CREMES, normally sold in stick form, offer the heaviest coverage and should be used primarily for hiding blemishes. Solid cremes are often used to minimize under-eye circles, but sometimes they're too thick for the delicate skin under the eye and actually make dark circles look worse by drawing attention to the area. Apply with a finger, or use a brush for a thinner application. Blend with a sponge. **TUBES** give creamier, lighter coverage, which can be further thinned by mixing with foundation (use a small brush). Oil-free formulations make them perfect for spot-covering pimples. **LIQUIDS IN A WAND** are ideal for covering problem areas and evening out skin tone. They blend easily into bare skin and can be used without a foundation if the color is right, providing quicker and slightly denser coverage than liquid foundation. They yield the lightest texture and are perfect for fast face repair. **PENCIL STICKS** cover tiny imperfections, like broken capillaries, because tiny flaws can be pinpointed without blending.

C O N C E A L E R

OUR FACES EXPOSE THE WAY WE LIVE. DARK UNDER-EYE CIRCLES, BROKEN CAPILLARIES, PIMPLES—THEY TATTLE ON OUR SLEEPING HABITS, WHAT WE EAT AND DRINK, HOW MUCH TIME WE'RE SPENDING WITH our skin exposed to the elements. Concealers help to cover imperfections and signs of life-style excess. Choose a color that's a shade lighter than your natural skin tone—one with a neutral undertone if you are fair-skinned, a yellowish tint if your skin is medium to olive-toned. As with foundation, avoid pinks and oranges. They will highlight what you'd rather hide.

HOW TO **EMERGENCY FIXES.** Because your foundation also conceals, concealer should go on after foundation. Sometimes it may turn out you don't need concealer at all. For dark eyes, consider applying a dot of concealer inside the corner of your eye. For **UNDER-EYE CIRCLES,** use a foundation brush to mix concealer with your foundation to ensure a perfect color match. Then dot with brush or finger underneath the eye, and lightly blend with a slightly damp sea sponge. **PIMPLES** can be covered by using a small brush and painting concealer directly over the blemish, or dotting it with a concealer pencil. Fade out edges with your fingertip. Apply powder directly over the concealed pimple to set. **BROKEN CAPILLARIES** can be traced with a concealer pencil if there are few of them, or covered with a creamy concealer for larger areas. They can also be treated surgically by cauterizing them with a tiny laser. Do not attempt this at home. **SCARS** are smooth and don't give concealer much to grab on to. Use a heavy creme concealer, then set with powder. **PUFFY EYES** are one thing that concealer can't conceal. Cold compresses applied to the area every five or ten minutes are more effective. More effective still is avoiding drinking too much fluid, especially caffeinated beverages, before you go to bed.

[S T E P **3.** P O W D E R]

MAKEUP WITHOUT POWDER IS FLEETING AT BEST. UNFORTUNATELY, POWDER IS THE FIRST THING MOST OF US SKIP WHEN WE'RE IN A HURRY. WE ALSO MIGHT WORRY THAT IT WILL LOOK CAKEY ON OUR SKIN.

We may think of it as old-fashioned, too. We are wrong. Powder is an absolute necessity for setting your foundation and concealer, as well as for prepping your skin so that you don't look like a Salvador Dali painting within an hour of putting on your makeup. Used by itself, powder gives skin a smoother, more polished look and minimizes pores. Pressed onto the eyelids with a latex wedge before applying liner and shadow, it allows eye makeup to sit better and last longer. And applied lightly after wiping away shiny, old makeup, powder is the ultimate touchup.

Powder puffs can cake your face with too much of a good thing and make it look heavy. Apply powder with a brush for a light, sheer finish, then use a latex wedge to press it on the area around the eyes and nose—this will help set eye makeup and slow down the shine on your nose. Loosening pressed powder with a brush, blowing off the excess, then dusting it over your face can give a lighter effect than using a compact pad.

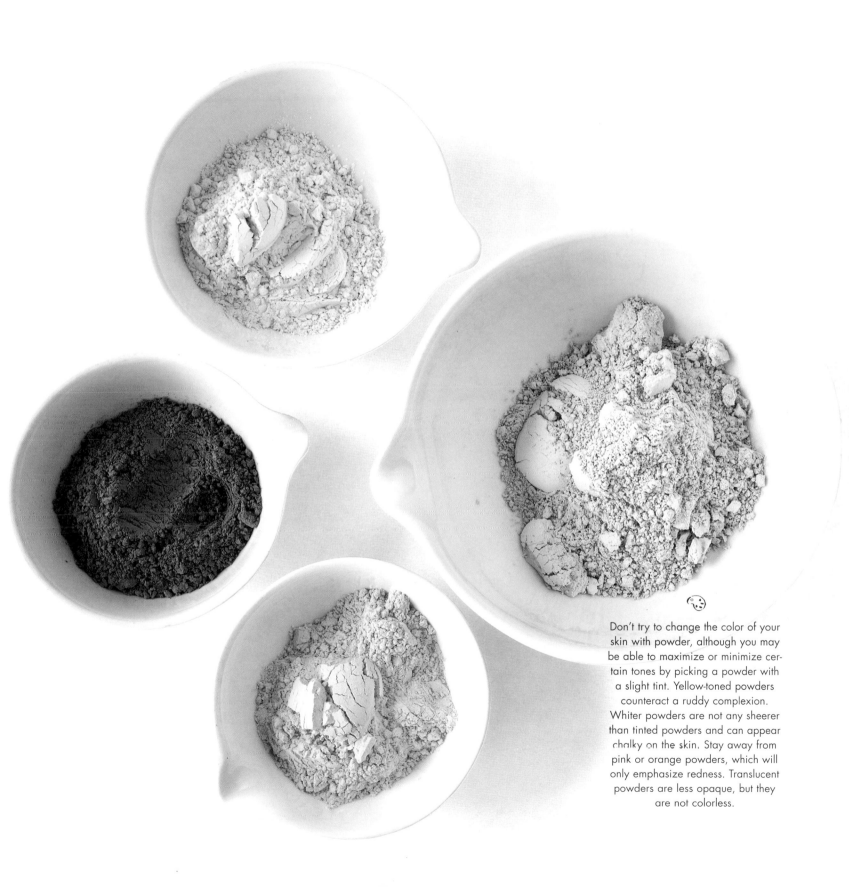

Don't try to change the color of your skin with powder, although you may be able to maximize or minimize certain tones by picking a powder with a slight tint. Yellow-toned powders counteract a ruddy complexion. Whiter powders are not any sheerer than tinted powders and can appear chalky on the skin. Stay away from pink or orange powders, which will only emphasize redness. Translucent powders are less opaque, but they are not colorless.

POWDER

Loose vs. pressed. Powder is lightest and most natural looking when it's used in its loose form. Loose powder is also available in a wider selection of colors than pressed, and can be custom blended. Use it instead of foundation to lightly even out your skin tone. Cut down on the shine of oily skin with an oil-free, matte formula. Add some sheen to dry skin by dabbing on a moisturizing, iridescent loose powder. The drawback is that if you're touching up makeup, it can be messy, and it's not the easiest thing to pop into an evening bag. Pressed powder is about convenience. It comes in compacts that travel well, but it lies more heavily on the face and can deaden a delicate, dry complexion. Apply with a pad or latex sponge for thicker coverage and quick T-zone touchups. Or loosen lightly with a brush, then dust on for the lighter look of loose powder. Look for an oil-free formula if your skin is oily or prone to breaking out, one with a moisturizer if you are worried about dryness.

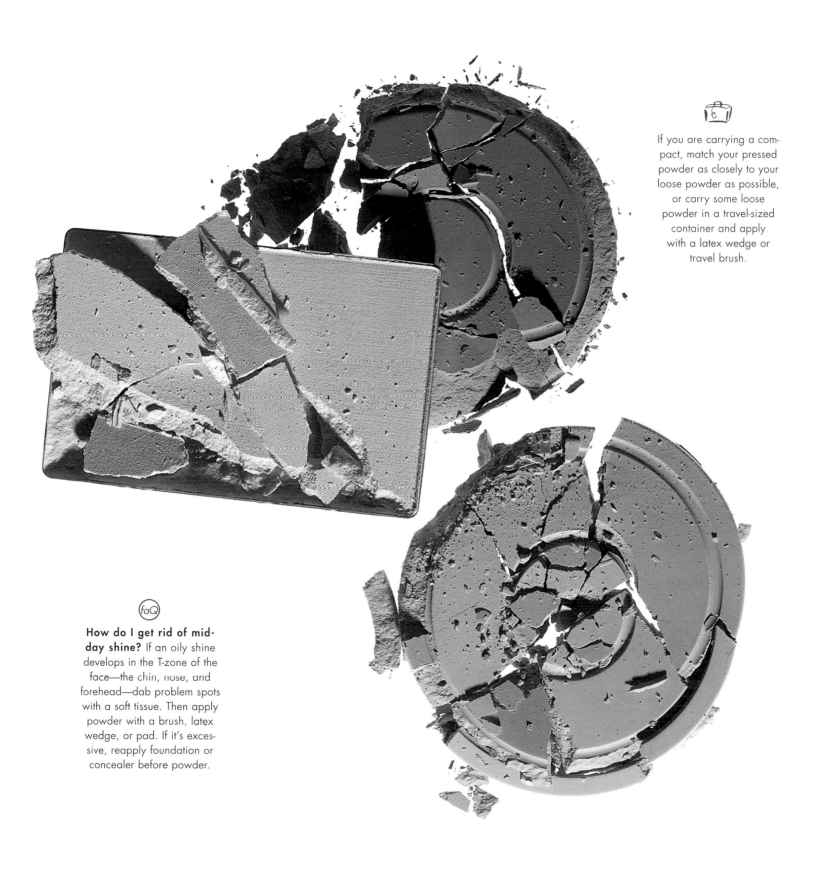

If you are carrying a compact, match your pressed powder as closely to your loose powder as possible, or carry some loose powder in a travel-sized container and apply with a latex wedge or travel brush.

faQ

How do I get rid of mid-day shine? If an oily shine develops in the T-zone of the face—the chin, nose, and forehead—dab problem spots with a soft tissue. Then apply powder with a brush, latex wedge, or pad. If it's excessive, reapply foundation or concealer before powder.

[S T E P **4.** B L U S H]

[blush]

IF YOU SEEK A HEALTHY-LOOKING GLOW, AS IF YOU'VE JUST

TAKEN A BRISK WALK, BLUSH CAN HELP. BUT HOW MUCH COLOR DO

YOU REALLY NEED? TOO MUCH OF IT AGES AN OLDER FACE AND LOOKS HARD ON A

younger one. A good blush should add subtle glow and gently shape your face. Apply it to the cheeks only. **Texture mix.** Blending a tinted moisturizer with a creme blush can create a fresh, dewy appearance and soft, muted color for drier and older skins.

What type of blush stays on the longest? That depends on your skin type. If you have dry skin, creme-based products will work well, while powder blush works well on oily skin.

Apply it all over your face, then dab creme blush on your cheeks and blend. Or mix tinted moisturizer and creme blush together on the back of your hand, then apply it to your cheeks. You'll soften the color of the blush and achieve a warm, translucent effect.

"She had rouged her cheeks to a color otherwise seen only on specially ordered Pontiac Firebirds."

GEORGE V. HIGGINS
on Diana Vreeland

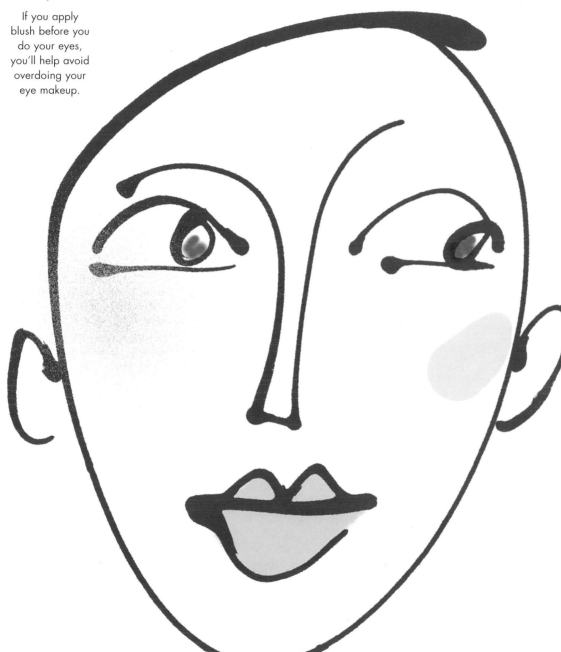

CREME BLUSH

Creme blushes go on like a creme and give a dewy finish, but they don't work well with oily skin or large pores. Applied with your fingers, they work particularly well on normal and dry skin. The effect is luminous, perfect for achieving a natural glow. Put on before adding powder. **POWDER BLUSH,** applied with a blush brush, gives a soft dusting of color that works well on all skin types. It's the most popular, because it's the easiest to use. If using on bare skin, apply loose powder first to prevent blotchiness. **GEL BLUSH** creates a sheer, translucent glow that is light enough to blend into bare skin. It's long-lasting, usually waterproof, and can even stand up to exercise. Rub into the cheeks with fingertips. Be careful, because gels tend to stain if spilled. They can be hard to blend, especially on dry skin. Apply them before adding powder.

[blushing]

Smile and find the apples of your cheeks. This is where you naturally blush. It is also the starting point for applying blush. Unless your face shape is obviously round, square, or long, just apply blush to the apples of the cheeks with a slight upward and outward motion. If you have an angular face, go light on the blush. Heavy blush will overemphasize sharp features and can look severe.

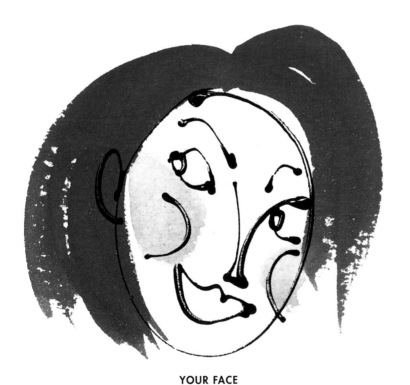

YOUR FACE

You can achieve subtle shaping with blush. The crimson rule: never brush it into your hairline.

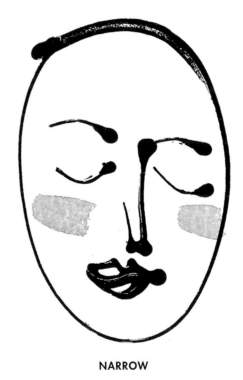

NARROW

For a wider appearance, start closer in on the apples and brush outward across the face.

Color. FAIR SKIN and lighter complexions look warmed up in soft, muted pinks with a hint of beige. MEDIUM SKIN can take even warmer pinks, with a brownish tint. OLIVE and YEL-LOW-TONED SKIN requires deeper brown-based shades with red, plum, and soft berry undertones to counter its natural yellowish cast. DARK SKIN looks best in rich colors, like cinnamon and nutmeg, and can glow under soft, deep bronze, cocoa, and red browns.

Face contouring. The use of brown-tinted cremes and powders on the sides of the face to create the effect of high cheekbones, or the layering of one blush color on top of another, is known as "face contouring" and looks artificial in everyday light. It should be applied by experts and confined to television appearances and professional photo shoots.

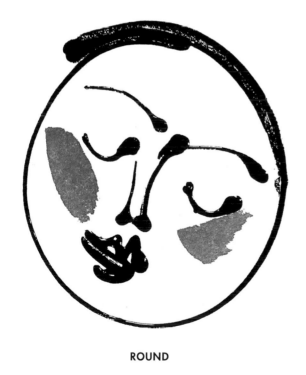

ROUND

Apply blush from the mid-apple of the cheeks and sweep it along the highest part of the cheekbone.

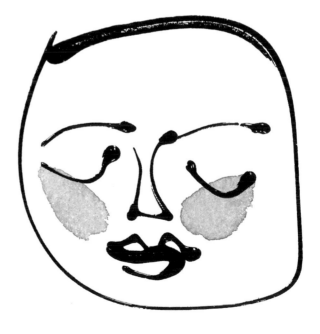

SQUARE

Use a light hand with the blush. Since you already have a strong bone structure, you don't need as much.

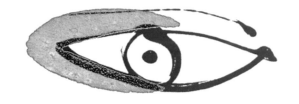

Eyes

YOU'VE HEARD IT BEFORE: IT'S ALL ABOUT THE EYES. INNOCENCE. GUILT. LOVE. HATRED. THE FIRST THING WE NOTICE IN A STRANGER'S FACE, THEY TRULY ARE WINDOWS INTO THE SOUL. SO HOW SHOULD WE dress them? Do we drape them with heavy lids and lashes? Is the wide-eyed delineation of a silent-film actress our style, or do we prefer the lighter, more natural look of a high school athlete? A smear of shadow or a gash of eyeliner can make our eyes appear farther apart, more deeply set, innocently wide, or sultrily half-shut. Iridescent shine brightens a young face. Eyes are about power and mystery, innocence and seduction. The makeup you use to transform them should follow the emotion you want your eyes to convey.

"Now you've seen me," she said calmly, "and I suppose you're about to say that my green eyes are burning into your brain."

F. SCOTT FITZGERALD, *This Side of Paradise*

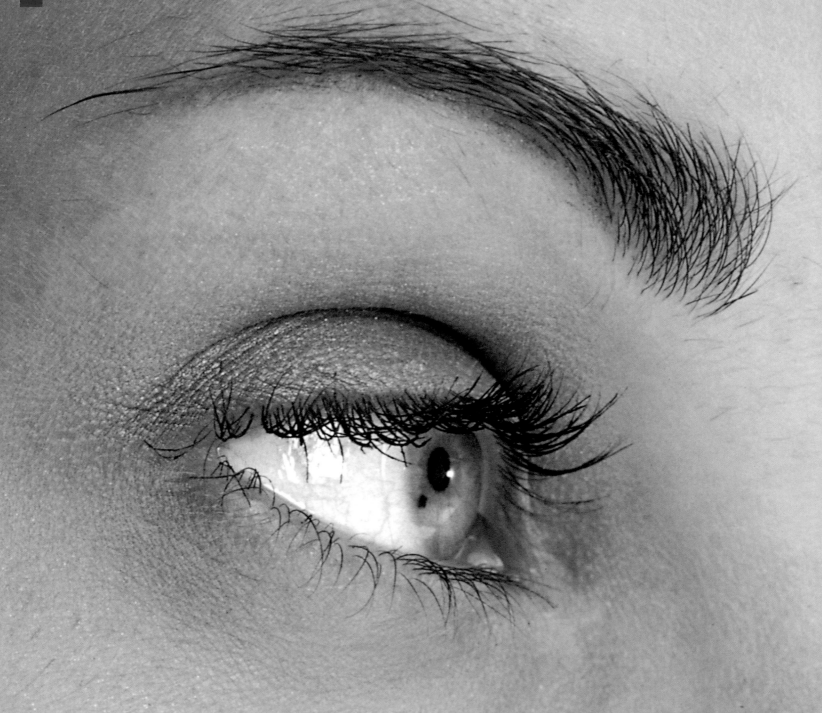

[🕮 EYEBROW PLUCKING *first aid—page 174*]

MOST OF US DON'T REALIZE THE IMPACT OUR BROWS HAVE

ON OUR OVERALL LOOK. BROODING LIKE BROOKE SHIELDS'S, OR ARCHED FOR HIGH HOLLYWOOD GLAMOUR, THEY FRAME AND BALANCE THE FACE. A WELL-GROOMED brow can make eyes appear larger and give your face the cheapest lift on the block. Brows are irresistibly changeable. You can't force a completely new shape into being, but you can fake some big effects. The best for you? Consider your style. If you prefer the look of thinner, more arched brows, great—but beware of creating the look of constant surprise overly rounded brows can create. If you like a natural brow, go light on the plucking and follow the line you already have—but remember that heavy brows close up the eyes and can overpower the rest of the face.

eyebrows

HOW TO Brows can be dyed—by a professional—or lightened slightly with a facial-hair bleach. Lighter brows make your features look softer and open up your face. Or you can fill them out yourself with makeup. Use a brow powder or fade in a brow pencil with a brow brush for the most natural look. Eyebrow pencils and powders are not the same as eye pencils and shadows. They are duller, drier, and more matte, so as not to coat the brow hairs in creamy, shiny colors. You can also brush shape into your brows, creating a smooth finish by brushing in the direction your hairs are growing, or separating the hairs for a more finished look. **COLOR.** In general, go for the browns, even if your brows are black. Fill in holes or create definition with a color similar to your own. If you are very fair, a slightly darker brow will give more definition. Blonde or light-brown brows look best with light brown. Redheads can use auburn shades. Brunette brows look good with dark brown tones; black hair demands them. **SHAPE.** If you're serious about changing the shape of your brows, go to a pro. If you just need a little cleanup, you can do it yourself. Stick with your natural line. Tidy up only the straggly hairs underneath. If necessary, clean up hairs between brows. Avoid plucking on top, as it can distort the natural shape. **UNRULY BROWS.** For long and curly eyebrows, brush them up, then snip individual long hairs unevenly for a natural look. For a soft sheen, apply petroleum jelly, then brush the brows into place. Or use brow gel or a spritz of hair spray on your brow brush for the same effect with greater hold.

 A clean eyebrow, plucked of straggling hairs, is the facial equivalent of a freshly laundered white shirt.

EYELINER

JEZEBEL AND CLEOPATRA HAD IT TOUGH, HAVING TO GRIND KOHL FROM A MIX OF BURNT ALMONDS AND THE ORES OF ANTIMONY, MANGANESE, AND LEAD. THE OPTIONS ARE NOW FAR SIMPLER THAN THEY WERE EVEN A DECADE AGO.

Use **CREAMY PENCILS**, for a strong defining line. Versatile **POWDER PENCILS** give an eyeshadow finish whether you're using them to line or to fade into a shadow. **FELT-TIP EYELINERS** don't smudge and last a long time, but their precise line can look severe on older eyes. **FAT CRAYONS**, with their creamy-powdered texture, double as shadow or liner for a soft, often shimmery

Should I apply eyeliner before eyeshadow?

If you apply eyeliner to your eyes first, your eyeshadow will soften the line, creating a more natural look.

effect. **LIQUID EYELINER** lets you brush on those Marilyn Monroe eyes, or use a wand for instant definition. Just make sure that any liner you use is not so hard that it tugs at your skin when you apply it. **Color.** Dark brown and black work well for pretty much everyone, but black is more dramatic, better saved for special occasions. Neutral tones—variations of brown, gray, charcoal, and black—are also classics.

 Chill your eye pencils before sharpening. They'll be less apt to break.

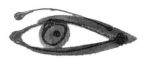

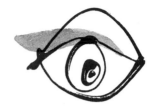

NARROW EYES can seem wider if you emphasize the outer portion of the top lid, lightly fading inward. They can also be opened up by lining underneath the eye with a thick, soft line.

CLOSE-SET EYES Definition goes at the outer corners of the eyes to draw attention outward.

LARGE, ROUND EYES can be shaped by lining the top lid and making the line slightly fatter at the outer corner of your eye.

 Eyeliner will have longer staying power if you apply a tiny bit of loose powder to your lid with a latex wedge before applying liner.

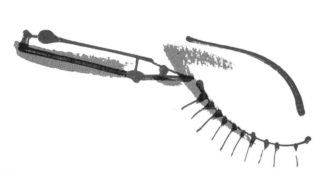

1. DEFINE. Line outer eye with pencil. Start from outside and work inward.

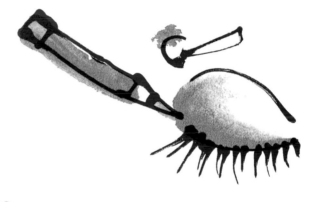

2. SOFTEN. Blend pencil with a sponge-tip applicator to soften and achieve a shadowing effect.

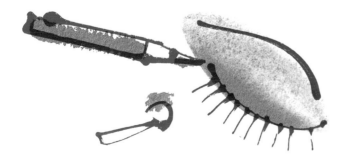

3. EMPHASIZE. Apply shadow over pencil with a sponge-tip applicator or an eyeshadow brush to soften.

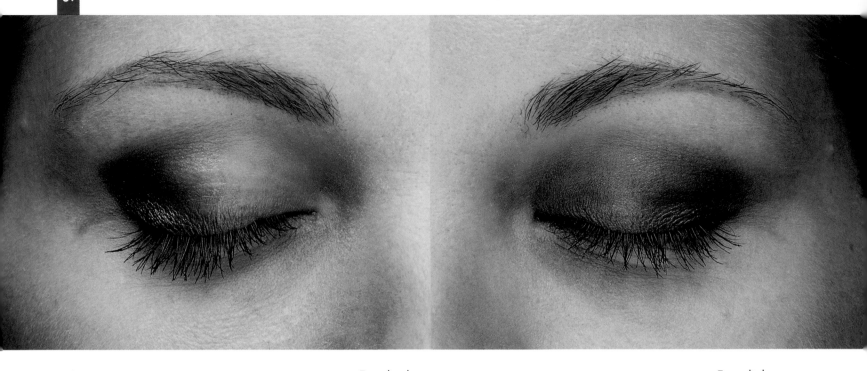

HIGH DEFINITION. For shadow, use a sponge-tip applicator for more precision and a more defined application. The emphasis is usually on the outside corner of the lid.

SOFT WASH. For a lighter touch, use a fluffy eyeshadow brush to apply a thin layer of shadow, with no specific definition.

HOW TO SMALL EYES. Light, shimmery, neutral tones can help open them up. Apply shadow over the lid and under the eye for a soft, smudgy effect. This will give more width to the eyes. **CLOSE-SET EYES.** Define only the outer corners to make eyes seem farther apart. **WIDE-SET EYES.** Make a narrow band of shadow all over your lids, from inner eye to outer, to give a greater sense of balance. **DEEP-SET EYES.** Light, pale shadows with a hint of shimmer highlight and open up the whole eye area. A little smudge of dark shadow at the outer corner helps define. **PROMINENT EYES.** Soft-pedal surprised-looking eyes by shading the upper lid with a darker shadow and extending it above the natural crease. Use a highlighting shadow only under the arch of the eyebrow to give them a lift. Pencil works best at the outer corners to lift **DROOPY EYELIDS.** A softer result can be achieved by applying a neutral yet darkish shadow at the outer corners of the eyes. Avoid color in the middle of the eye.

EYESHADOW

MARLENE DIETRICH SCULPTED HER SMOLDERING GLANCE BY LIGHTING A MATCH UNDER A SAUCER TO MAKE CARBON, WHICH SHE THEN MIXED WITH BABY OIL AND SMEARED INTO A SHADOW THAT STARTED JUST

above her lashes and faded away toward the outside of her eyebrow. Whether eyeshadow is about definition or soft focus, its purpose is to bring out your baby blues, or browns, or hazels, or greens. Are you an Ivory Girl? A pale, shimmering wash over the whole eyelid gives a quiet, natural look. Cruella DeVille? Darker tones paint your eyes into high drama. Eyeshadow colors can be soft and neutral, or bright and intense. Choose textures that suit you. While iridescence looks pretty, the shine emphasizes wrinkles. Older eyes should stick with matte or satin textures that glide on smoothly. **Warm and cool.** With eyeshadow, you want a shade that contrasts with your eye color to help bring out your eyes. "Cool" eyeshadow shades include gray, blue, purple, and green. They look good with darker eyes. "Warm" shades, which are basically variations on browns, look better with lighter eyes.

"Don't it make my brown eyes blue?"

CRYSTAL GAYLE

EYELASHES

EYELASHES MAY HAVE THE PRACTICAL PURPOSE OF KEEPING DEBRIS OUT OF OUR EYES, BUT WE'VE invested them with much deeper meaning. We hold our lashes in such reverence that we bat them for attention, and even make wishes on them when they fall out. Still, most of us have complaints. Our lashes are too short, too pale, too sparse, or too straight. So naturally we turn to mascara and the eyelash curler to draw attention to our eyes and make them appear larger.

HOW TO

MASCARA. Its application should be your last makeup step, so that powder doesn't dull your lashes. Apply a mascara wand to the base of your lashes and wiggle it horizontally for a few seconds. Then lift the wand up and out to the tips of your lashes. Let your lashes dry before applying a second coat, and don't apply more than two coats.

CURLERS. If your eyelashes don't curl up, eyelash curlers should help them look more noticeable. Before applying mascara, clamp a clean eyelash curler onto your lashes (without pulling) for 5 to 10 seconds.

FAKES. Long and thick, they recall the mods of the 1960s. Shorter and full, they can be used to define the shape of your eyes. A couple of single lashes can enhance by filling out your natural set. It's all in the gluing. Dot a thin line of eyelash glue along your upper lid. Slide the fakes into place along the tops of your own lashes, and press them gently along the base. If the glue dries white, cover with mascara or eyeliner.

COLOR. Fair lashes look most natural in brown mascara, although black can be worn for drama. Darker lashes look great in black mascara, although a deep brown gives a softer effect. Mascaras in olive, blue, and purple are for trendy looks. Clear mascara gives shine and curl to lashes that are naturally dark and curly. **FORMULA.** Thickening mascara coats each individual eyelash from shaft to tip. Lengthening mascara contains plastic polymers that cling just to the tips of your lashes, making them look longer. If your mascara wears off too quickly, try a long-lasting formula. Waterproof mascara is heavier and harder to remove than other formulas, making it a good choice for heavy-duty water activities but a poor choice for everyday wear. Pump the wand to mix the active ingredients. With all other types of mascara, it is a mistake to pump the wand because it can dry out the formula and spread bacteria contamination faster. Water-resistant mascara is a lighter formula recommended for weddings and screenings of *Now, Voyager*. **SHAPE.** Choose your mascara as much for the brush as for the formula. Bristles should be far enough apart to avoid clumping but close enough to ensure coverage. A wand with shorter, thinner bristles yields a lighter coat of mascara. Denser bristles hold more mascara, for a heavier coat.

"Your eyelashes sparkle like gilded grass."
LIZ PHAIR, *"Supernova"*

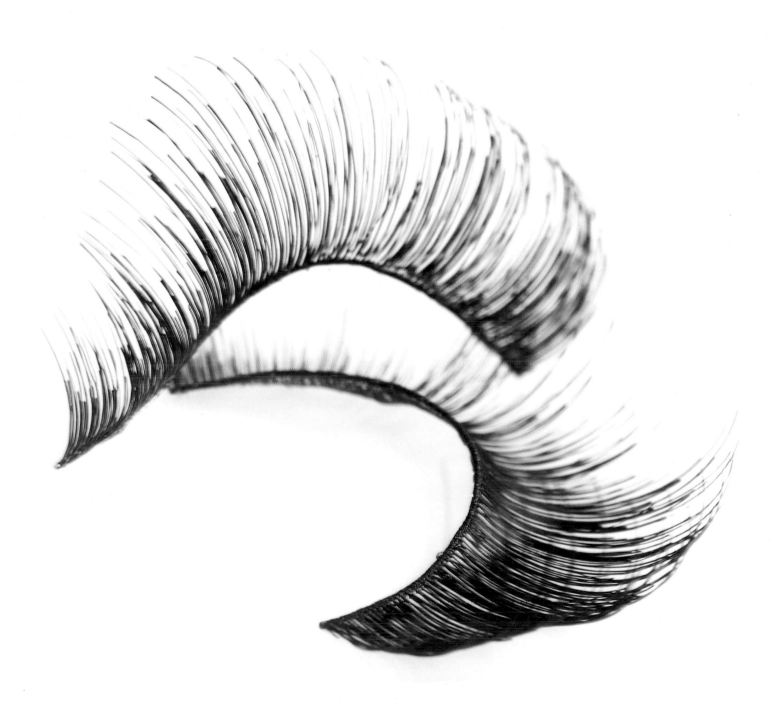

MORE mascara.

MASCARA FIRST BECAME FAMOUS IN 1915, AFTER

T. L. WILLIAMS SAW HIS SISTER MABEL RUBBING PETROLEUM JELLY

INTO HER LASHES "TO MAKE THEM HEALTHY AND MORE NOTICEABLE." NAMING HIS

company after his sister, Williams put out Lash Brow Line at 25 cents a shot. Later,

mascaras in France were inspired by the pomade Napoleon III used to groom his mus-

tache. Long used to add mystery and allure to the eyes, mascara in its modern-day

forms can itself be mystifying. But where there are questions, there are answers.

Don't throw out your old mascara wand. Clean it with eye-makeup remover and use it to declump lashes.

Should I put mascara on the bottom lashes as well? If you are wearing eyeliner on your upper and lower lids, then you can put mascara on both top and bottom. But if your lower lid is unlined, mascara can look spidery on your lower lashes. Stick with the upper lashes only. **To touch up for evening, can I apply a new coat over my old mascara?** Yes, but apply it with a light touch to prevent clumping. **How can I avoid runny mascara?** If it's simply a matter of having teary eyes, then a waterproof or water-resistant mascara will help. Otherwise, try applying powder to lashes before mascara. If around the eyes skin is very oily, mascara may run, so powder the skin. **What is the quickest way to get smudged mascara off my skin?** Moisten a cotton swab and wipe away smudges as quickly as possible. If the smudge has dried, dip the swab in makeup remover and try again. **Do eyelashes grow back?** Sometimes they do, sometimes they don't. Eyelashes can become brittle for reasons ranging from poor diet to bad cleaning habits. **Will it harm my lashes to wear mascara every day?** No, as long as you clean your lashes properly at night. **What are signs that mascara has gone bad?** Mascara has a shelf life of about two or three months. After that, it becomes dry and clumpy, and can be unhygienic. To preserve mascara, never pump the wand unless you're using a waterproof formula. Pumping dries out the formula and increases the air and bacteria content, both of which will speed up degeneration. **My eyes water when I wear mascara. What can I do?** Look for fiber-free mascaras, or simply try curling lashes and applying a little petroleum jelly to help your lashes appear thicker and longer. **What should I look for in a mascara wand?** Bristles that are too close will clump your mascara, but if they're too far apart, you won't get enough coverage. Look for a brush no more than a half-inch wide, and avoid curved models: it's easier to reach angles and corners with a straight wand. **What's the best way to take care of my lashes?** Always remove all traces of eye makeup before going to bed. If you don't, aside from looking like a prizefighter when you wake up, you risk drying your lashes, causing them to break, which can even be bad for your eyes. Use products especially designed for the job. Wipe until a pad or cotton ball comes away clean. There are also eyelash balms that condition lashes at night. Look for a conditioning mascara with provitamin B_5 or polymers in it.

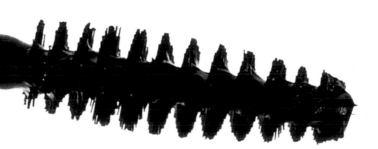

Lips

"DON'T GIVE ME ANY OF YOUR LIP," WE MIGHT SAY WHEN SOMEONE'S PUTTING ON AN ATTITUDE WE DON'T APPRECIATE. ATTITUDE IS, AFTER ALL, WHAT LIPS ARE ALL ABOUT. THEY CAN BE PALE AND INNOCENT OR pouty and seductive, and with the right lipstick, you're in the driver's seat. Suffice it to say, we like our lips moist and plump, and sometimes we like them red. **Texture.** It's as important as color. MATTE lipsticks deliver intense color with no shine. They are drying, but they last longer than other formulas. CREME lipsticks also pack a good color punch and are more emollient than mattes. Lips look moist but not shiny. GLOSSY lip color usually comes in a wand, tube, or tub and is the least drying. Its sheer colors do not stay on long, but they look fresh and natural.

 PROTECTION The skin on the lips is thinner and lower in melanin than the skin on the rest of the face, so it's important to protect your lips from sun, wind, and cold. Put balm on your lips before putting on any other makeup, then dab them lightly with your fingertip just before applying lipstick. Wear clear balm over your lip pencil for a nourishing, lightly tinted gloss.

1. Use foundation as a concealer, applying it minimally only where needed, to retain the natural glow of the skin.

2. Lightly powder face.

3. Lightly brush cheeks with a sheer almond-rose blush.

4. Define eyes with a soft brown lining pencil at the outer corners, then blend with a sponge-tip applicator for a soft effect.

5. Use brown mascara for soft definition.

6. Brush a soft brownish-mauve lip color lightly over the lips for a subtle finish.

Lips

HOW TO Puckering your lips when you're applying **LIPSTICK** scrunches up your coloring surface and may make you miss a few spots. Stretch your lips, then apply color, to ensure better coverage. **LIP LINERS** help to define your lips and make lipstick stay on longer and better. They help to prevent color bleeding and give you a guideline to follow when applying lipstick. They are essential for older lips, which can become pale and lose their natural lip line. **LIP BALM** keeps lips conditioned. Applied before lip color, it smooths lips and primes them for the lipstick. And applied on top of lip color, it glosses up a matte texture. A **LIP BRUSH** can give you a more precise finish and a thinner application. **Lip etiquette. TO AVOID COATING YOUR TEETH WHEN YOU SMILE,** apply lipstick, then insert your index finger into your mouth. Close your lips lightly around it, and pull out your finger. Consider, briefly, changing your name to Luscious. **TO KEEP LIPSTICK OFF THE RIM OF YOUR COFFEE MUG,** try a

How can I make my lipstick last longer?

After applying lipstick, blot your lips, then reapply and blot again. Your lipstick will have twice the staying power. You can also powder your lips or apply foundation to them before putting on lipstick, but this may dry them. Lining your lips also helps hold lipstick in place.

long-lasting formula, or blot your lipstick carefully after adding a new coat. **TOUCHING UP IN PUBLIC** is fine: if you're comfortable doing it, Emily Post will back you up. But at a business lunch, it may be considered too feminine a gesture. **Lip shapes. FULL LIPS** a problem? Hard to believe. But too much of a good thing can be toned down by using softer, sheerer colors, without liner. Color should be focused in the middle of the mouth, then bled out to the edges. Cherry red lips require sheer, soft colors to avoid looking too intense. **THIN LIPS** can look mean-mouthed under dark, hard lip color. Lighter, sheerer colors and gloss will make lips look fuller. Lip liner should not be used outside the natural lip line in an attempt to make thin lips appear fuller. Instead, outline at the extreme edge of lips in a liner that is the same color as your lipstick. By extending the line of your lips all the way to the corners of the mouth, lips can be made to appear bigger. Lip liner can be used to even out **CROOKED LIPS** by lining in symmetry.

> "Where lipstick is concerned, the important thing is not the color, but to accept God's final decision on where your lips end."
>
> **JERRY SEINFELD**

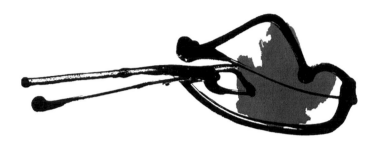

You can correct color mistakes or create a custom color by blending a top coat of lighter-colored lipstick into a too-dark shade. To subdue a bright color, blend on a top coat of darker color.

For precise, **LUSTROUS LIPS,** first coat a lip brush with lipstick. Then apply by starting in the middle of your mouth, holding the brush flat, and pull color to the edges of your lip, thinning as you move away from the center. If your lips are too glossy, dab them lightly with the pad of your finger.

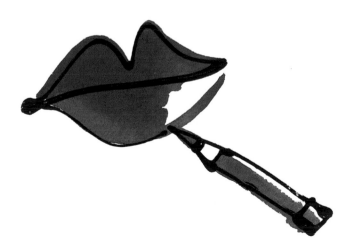

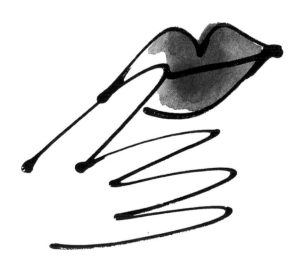

For **PURE COLOR,** put lipstick on straight from the stick and blot once with a tissue. Lining and coloring in your lips with a lip pencil gives a similar effect but can be drying.

Add **SHIMMER** to your basic color with an opalescent gloss. Or try plain old lip balm dabbed over the top lip and center of the bottom lip for a similar shimmering effect.

beauty

1. Apply makeup in daylight, near a window. It will look much more natural. If you don't have a window or it's dark outside, you can purchase at specialty stores lightbulbs specifically designed for makeup application. [page 108]

2. Update your makeup seasonally, even if it means just two new shades of lipstick. Your look will stay fresh and modern. [page 80]

3. Keep your makeup brushes clean. Wash them weekly [page 166], or they'll dry out and won't spread makeup evenly; worse, germs may accumulate.

4. Read fashion and beauty magazines for tips and updates on new products. Experiment.

5. Give your skin a break from makeup at least once a week. More important, accept your face without makeup and know you look fine. [page 17]

6. Don't skimp on quality when buying tools. [page 104]

7. Be gentle and never pull on your skin when applying makeup. [page 104]

8. Apply lip balm every morning and night for smooth, moist lips. [page 136]

9. Always apply loose powder immediately after putting on foundation and before adding the rest of your makeup. [page 113]

beast

1. Sleeping with your makeup on. Mascaraed lashes can break. Left-on foundations and blush can clog pores and cause breakouts.

2. Keeping makeup that you haven't used in years. If you get rid of it, not only will you finally be able to find the aspirin in the middle of the night, but you'll feel more in control of your daily makeup regimen. And all makeup has a shelf life. [page 167]

3. Sticking with the same makeup look indefinitely. Maybe it once worked, but nothing lasts forever. You change, and so does makeup technology. [page 95] And no one looks older than someone stuck in time.

4. Picking an eyeshadow color that's the same color as your eyes. The monochromatic look won't enhance them.

5. Overtweezing your eyebrows. If your eyebrows are too thin, your eyes will lose dimension, and you'll throw off the balance of your face. [page 127]

6. Wearing too much makeup. It can overpower, and attract more attention than you.

7. Putting foundation all over your face, up to your hairline. You'll look like you're wearing a mask. [page 113]

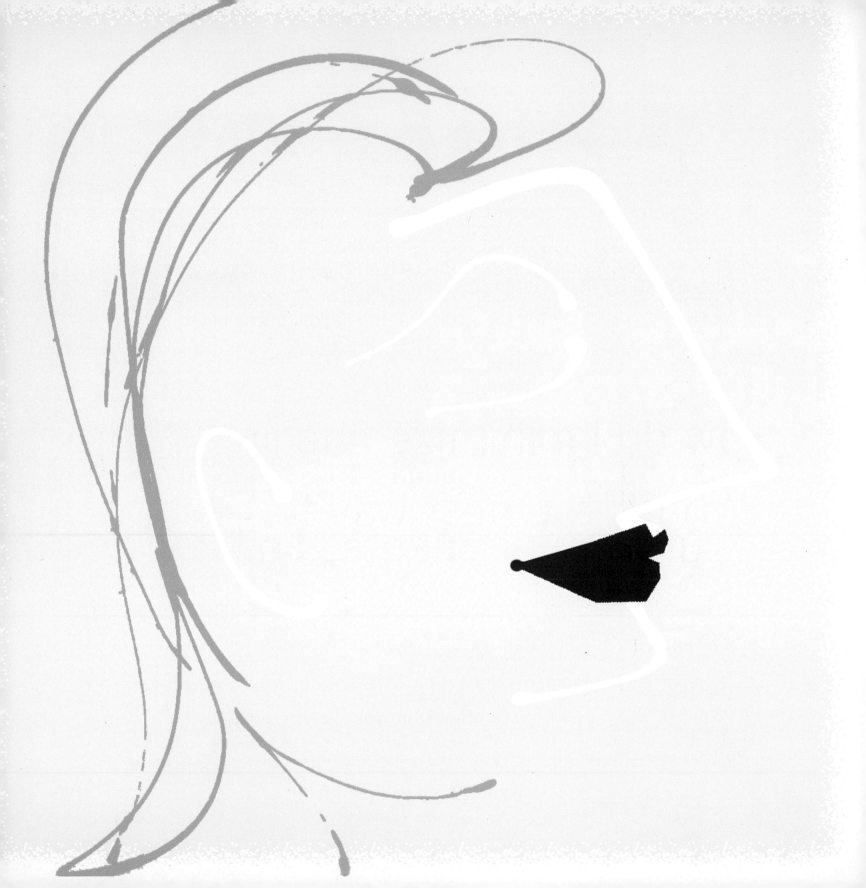

Looking Your Best

"She must redesign the face, smooth the anxious brows, separate the crushed eyelashes, wash off the traces of secret interior tears, accentuate the mouth as upon a canvas, so it will hold its luxuriant smile."

ANAÏS NIN
A Spy in the House of Love

FEELING PRETTY

You've figured it all out. You know what your skin type is, so you understand how to care for it. Makeup-wise, you know the colors, textures, and formulas your skin demands, and you know just when and how you want to wear them. You're enhancing, experimenting, or just touching up. What's left? Real-life application of everything you've learned—not just about skin care, powder, and paint, but about yourself.

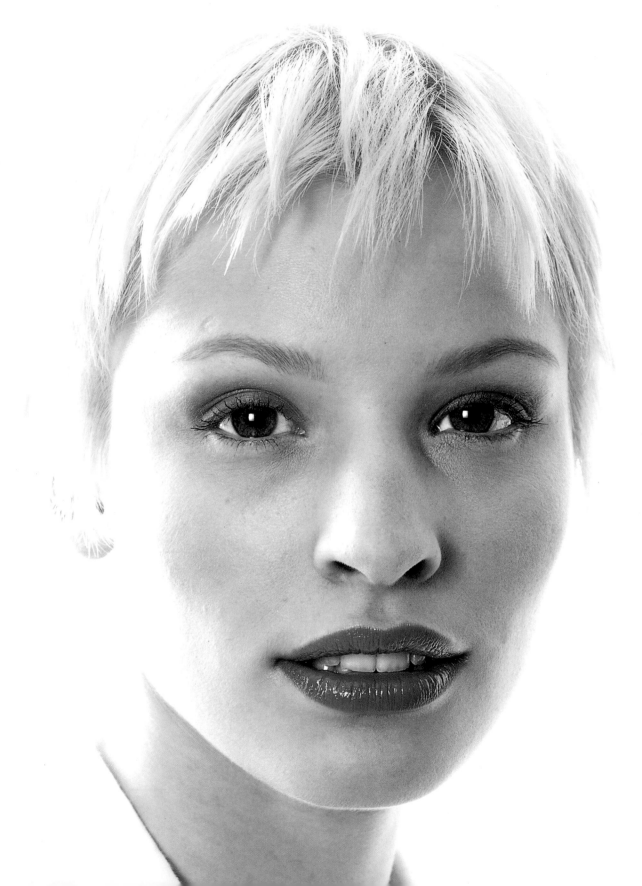

1. Apply a light liquid foundation with a slight yellow undertone.

2. Dust with a light-colored loose powder.

3. Add blush in a muted, barely there shade of pink.

4. In keeping with soft makeup, don't use eye-liner.

5. Apply a wash of warm brown eyeshadow all over the eyelid, with no specific definition.

6. Coat dark-brown mascara on upper lashes only.

7. Apply glossy pink-brown lip color to add natural subtlety.

BLONDE

LIGHT SKIN TENDS TO BE FRAGILE, EXISTING AT THE MERCY OF THE ELEMENTS. SUN AND WIND CAN CAUSE REDNESS AND PREMATURE WRINKLING—BOTH IMPORTANT FACTORS IN CHOOSING THE color and texture of your makeup. Determining your exact skin tone—and, therefore, the perfect foundation shade—can be difficult. Light skin can be very thin and bluish in color, or it can be reddish, from sun exposure and broken capillaries. It can even have faintly yellow undertones. But the overall effect is that you are pale. A pale face usually needs a little definition all over, especially on the lashes. Or you can go with simple drama: Keep the background light, and emphasize a single feature. Most of all, concentrate on keeping things fresh and warm.

FOUNDATION AND POWDER. Paler complexions do not support heavy makeup as well as darker ones, so think about a lighter, more liquid base formulation and loose powder. **LIPS.** Soft, warm pinks with mauve or brown undertones look pretty and understated, while something darker, like a deep, plummy red, can be a knockout for evening. A sheer gloss can be the perfect foil for dramatic eyes. **EYES.** Black mascara and pencil on the eyes looks great with nothing but a sheer, light lip color. Otherwise, keep eyeshadow natural and soft. **BROWS.** If you have light eyebrows, define your eyes and help frame your face by adding definition with a light-brown brow pencil and filling in lightly. **CHEEKS.** A little color goes a long way on pale skin. Keep blush soft and delicate by going only a few shades darker than your natural skin tone. Pinks with golden, peachy tones look best. Or, if you have it, let your own high cheek color shine through.

B L A C K

BLACK SKIN INCLUDES SUCH A HUGE RANGE OF SKIN TONES THAT IT'S NEARLY IMPOSSIBLE to make generalizations about makeup. It can be as light as olive skin or it can be ebony. Lighter-brown skin has a yellowish undertone, while darker-brown has a combination of yellow and mahogany tones. Finding the right foundation is the toughest assignment. It should not have any pink tones or contain too much titanium dioxide, which can cast an ashy wash over dark skin. It can be moisturizing or oil-free, depending on your skin type, although you should not confuse shiny skin with oily skin: your skin is oily only if you break out frequently. Dark skin does not tend to have the same problems with dryness as lighter skin, but that doesn't mean it's oily. It reflects light differently, giving off a kind of luminosity. Don't try to strip this away with harsh astringents. Excess shine can be controlled by using oil-free bases and powder.

HOW TO **FOUNDATION.** Look at brands that specialize in colors for black skin. They are usually better. Generally, avoid colors that are too red. Deep yellow tones work well for the vast range of black skin tones. **CHEEKS.** Warm light-brown peach-to-cinnamon tones in light, translucent textures make for soft definition on dark skin. **EYES.** Shimmery beiges and deep browns like copper, bronze, and mahogany bring out your eyes in a subtle way. The key is a sheer texture that allows the natural glow of black skin to shine through. Metallics complement the natural luminosity of dark skin in a way that is both striking and natural. Look for inky-black mascaras that are specially formulated to coat curly lashes smoothly. **LIPS.** Lips look great in deep berry shades—dark plum, blackberry, and burgundy are much more flattering than garish reds. Nude pinks and beiges are soft and pretty, but anything orange will clash with the yellow undertones of dark skin and will make you look washed out. Mocha, coffee, chocolate—any shade of brown—looks stunning. **HYPERPIGMENTATION.** Uneven pigmentation is to darker skin what broken capillaries and dark circles are to lighter skin: something to camouflage. Test foundation first on your face where you are lightest, and then again next to a darker patch of skin. Choose a color that is in between your lightest and your darkest coloring.

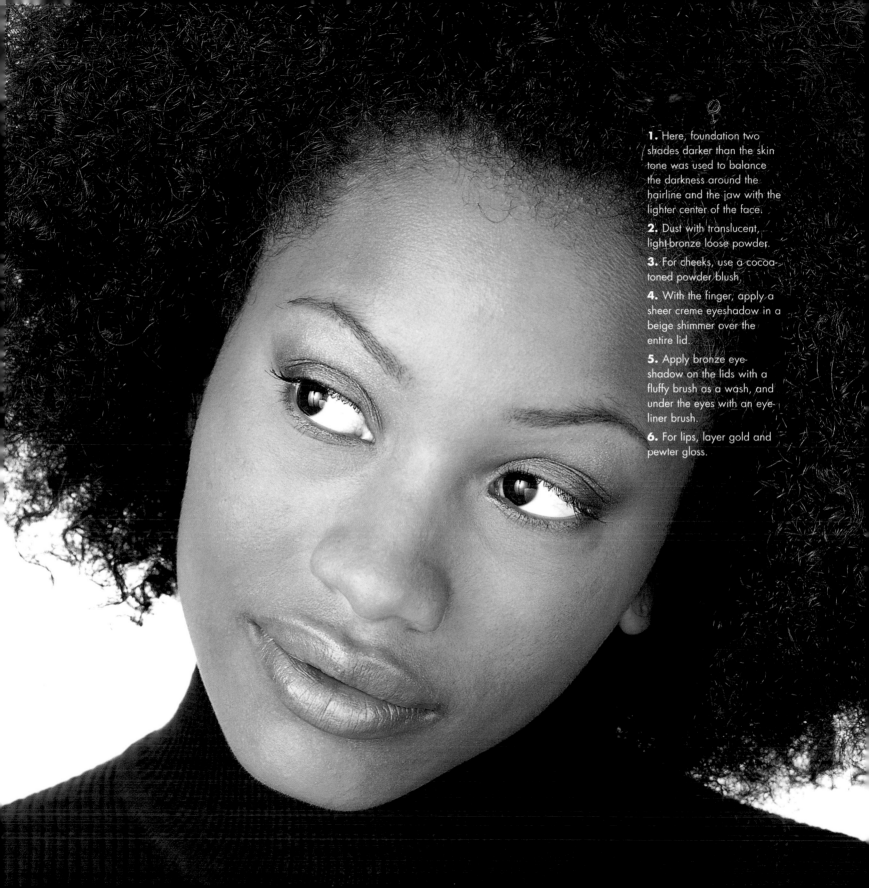

1. Here, foundation two shades darker than the skin tone was used to balance the darkness around the hairline and the jaw with the lighter center of the face.

2. Dust with translucent, light-bronze loose powder.

3. For cheeks, use a cocoa-toned powder blush.

4. With the finger, apply a sheer creme eyeshadow in a beige shimmer over the entire lid.

5. Apply bronze eye-shadow on the lids with a fluffy brush as a wash, and under the eyes with an eye-liner brush.

6. For lips, layer gold and pewter gloss.

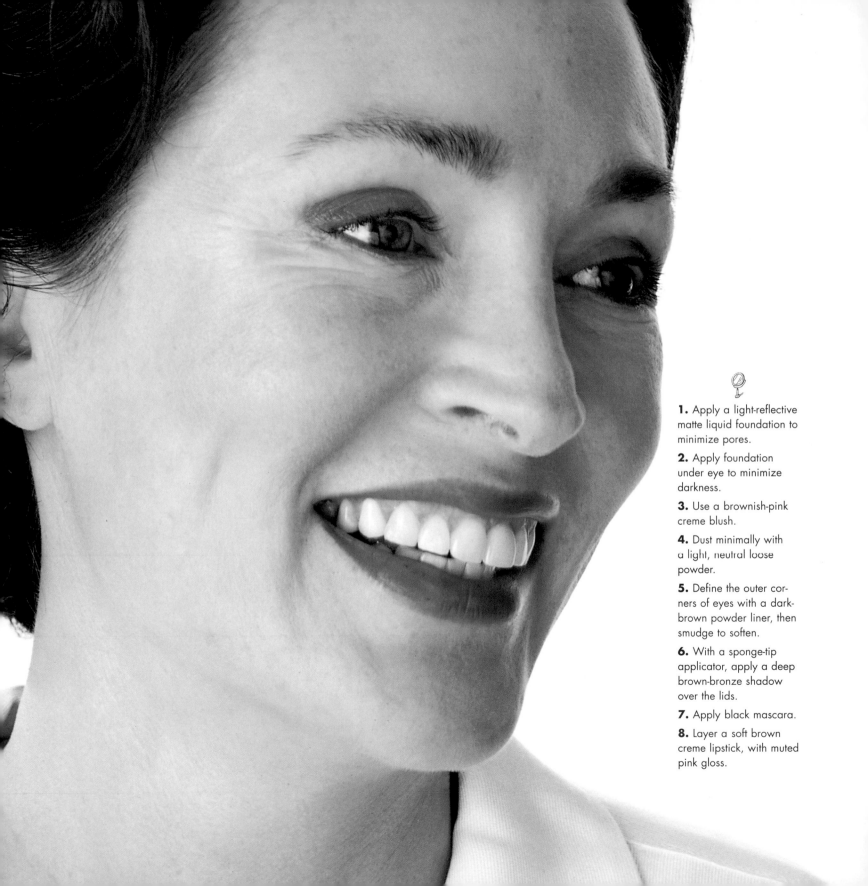

1. Apply a light-reflective matte liquid foundation to minimize pores.

2. Apply foundation under eye to minimize darkness.

3. Use a brownish-pink creme blush.

4. Dust minimally with a light, neutral loose powder.

5. Define the outer corners of eyes with a dark-brown powder liner, then smudge to soften.

6. With a sponge-tip applicator, apply a deep brown-bronze shadow over the lids.

7. Apply black mascara.

8. Layer a soft brown creme lipstick, with muted pink gloss.

MATURE

ONE MORNING YOU WAKE UP AND REALIZE THAT YOUR FACE HAS CHANGED. THE LINES AROUND YOUR MOUTH ARE MORE PROMINENT; YOU CATCH A GLIMPSE OF YOUR REFLECTION WHILE YOU'RE LAUGHING

and are startled by the laugh lines around your eyes. This makes you stop laughing and notice the worry lines on your forehead. Broken capillaries may lend a rosy hue to your cheeks and nose. Your face is in a state of transition. Years of living are now leaving their mark. Your well-earned wisdom and joys have combined with the effects of spending time outdoors and plain old everyday gravity to provide this newest version of

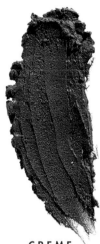

CREME BLUSH
adds a soft, creamy glow to mature skin.

you. It's at this point that some start to consider plastic surgery. Others shrug it off. Whatever you choose, your makeup must adapt to these changes as well. The colors, textures, and placement of makeup can enhance your features in the best possible way. The worst thing you can do is not adapt, and try to stick with the regimen you used when you had a different face. The results will make you look even older.

HOW TO **FOUNDATION.** Up to now, you may have gotten away with wearing no foundation. Now may be the time to start. A small amount can work wonders. Use foundation the same way you'd use a concealer: under eyes, around the nose, a little on the cheeks. Avoid textures that are too matte, which can emphasize wrinkles. A light-reflective foundation will minimize lines and give your skin a luminous quality. **CONCEALER.** Avoid using concealer under your eyes unless absolutely necessary. The heaviness of the product will settle there and emphasize lines. Instead, apply a little foundation there, with a flat brush to ensure a thinner application and lighter coverage. **BLUSH.** Sometimes mature skin can be dry and flaky. Look for a soft creme blush (not too bright) for a fresher, more dewy finish. **EYES.** Skip overly creamy eye pencils and shimmery eyeshadows. They tend to smudge and emphasize lines. Instead, choose powder-based pencils. They're softer, blend more easily, and run a lot less. **LIPS.** Color on lips—in natural shades as well as deep tones—can give your skin a real lift. Light pastels don't usually work as well, especially when contrasted with an uneven skin tone. Consider using a lip pencil for more definition if your lip line is getting weaker.

O L D E R

THERE IS NO SUCH THING AS AGE REVERSAL. YOU MAY CHOOSE TO FIGHT IT WITH CREAMS OR SCALPELS. You exercise and eat right. And then you age anyway. The skin on your face lightens in color and gets drier. It loses its elasticity and luster. Spidery lines appear around your eyes and mouth. Your lips become paler, thinner, and less defined. Just as your wardrobe changes with the years, so should your makeup. Dated makeup ages you faster than any indignity Mother Nature throws your way. Older beauty is about owning up to who you are, not hiding behind who you wish you were. It's about acceptance. Take a long, hard look at yourself, and wear your age proudly. The simple truth is that you may depend on makeup more now, but need less of it.

SHIMMERY LIQUID BASE adds light to your face. Lightly dab it, over foundation, on your cheek and brow bones. Or mix it with your foundation to give your skin a soft, delicate sheen. It will make your face look younger and more vibrant, and works with all skin colors.

HOW TO

FOUNDATION. Your skin has changed, so you need a new foundation. Look for a base that is light-reflective. For smooth, luminous coverage that won't emphasize lines, try a silicone-based product. Drier skin can be kept from flaking with a built-in moisturizer. **POWDER.** It won't dry out your skin, but to ensure that it sits lightly and smoothly on your skin, look for a very fine loose powder, with a moisturizing component. **BLUSH.** You want to restore a glow to your cheeks and subtly shape your face. Creme-formula blushes can give dry older skin a fresh, dewy look. Gels may stain older skin. **EYES.** Your lids may be wrinkled and have a bluish-red tone. Avoid strong colors and iridescent eyeshadows. Try muted neutrals, like brownish grays and soft browns. Mascara and eye pencil may be more important now than ever. Keep them soft, but use them to define your eyes and frame your face. **LIPS.** Matte lipsticks can be drying and emphasize lines, while high-gloss lipsticks can bleed and highlight wrinkles. Stick with creamy textures in rich colors that go with your skin tone. Too dark or vibrant a lipstick can harden and age your face. But shades that are too soft can make you look washed out. Lip liner is crucial to define faded lips and keep lipstick from bleeding. To further prevent lipstick from bleeding into the lines around your mouth, brush a little foundation around the outside of your lips and set with powder. Then apply color. If you want a hint of gloss, dab it in the middle of your lips, over your lip color.

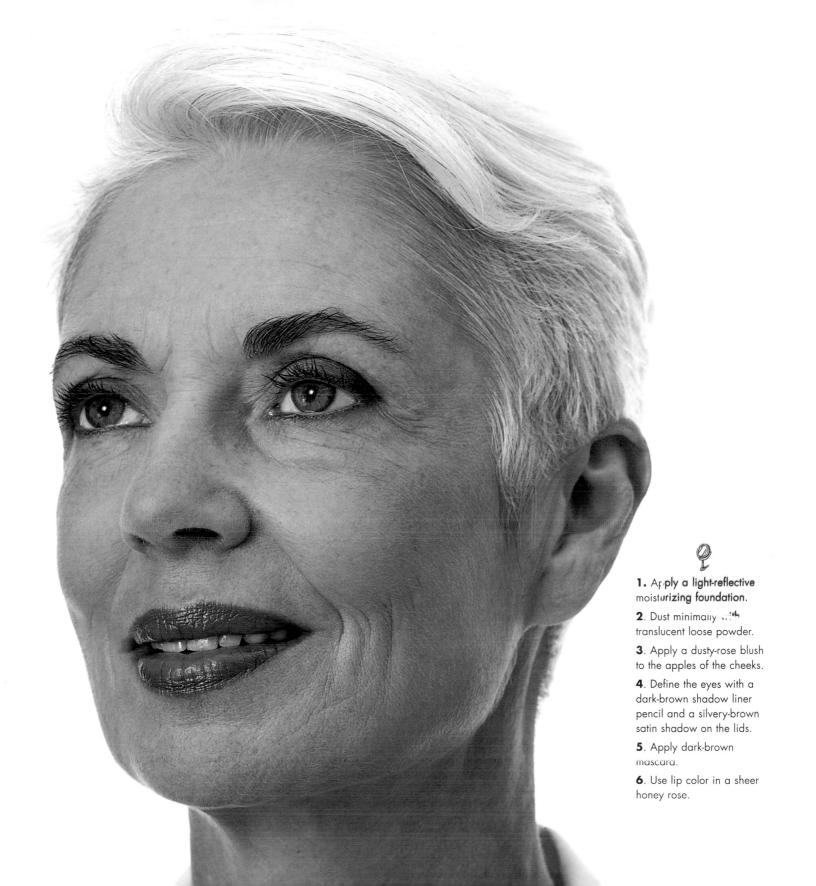

1. Apply a **light-reflective** moisturizing foundation.

2. Dust minimally with translucent loose powder.

3. Apply a dusty-rose blush to the apples of the cheeks.

4. Define the eyes with a dark-brown shadow liner pencil and a silvery-brown satin shadow on the lids.

5. Apply dark-brown mascara.

6. Use lip color in a sheer honey rose.

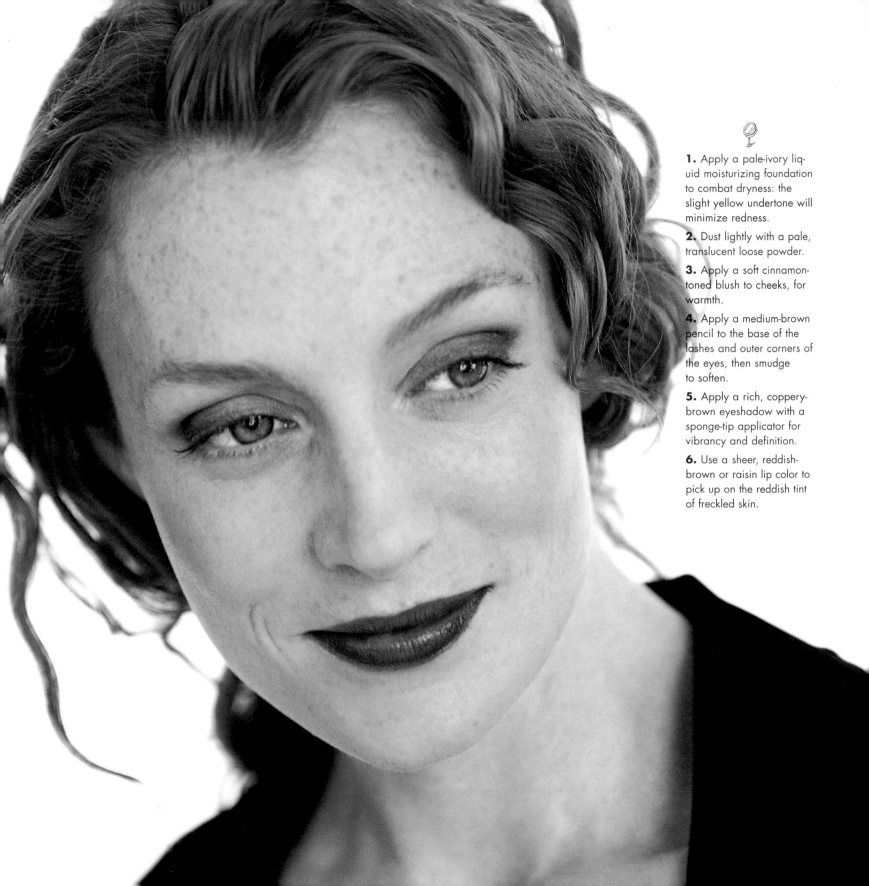

1. Apply a pale-ivory liquid moisturizing foundation to combat dryness: the slight yellow undertone will minimize redness.

2. Dust lightly with a pale, translucent loose powder.

3. Apply a soft cinnamon-toned blush to cheeks, for warmth.

4. Apply a medium-brown pencil to the base of the lashes and outer corners of the eyes, then smudge to soften.

5. Apply a rich, coppery-brown eyeshadow with a sponge-tip applicator for vibrancy and definition.

6. Use a sheer, reddish-brown or raisin lip color to pick up on the reddish tint of freckled skin.

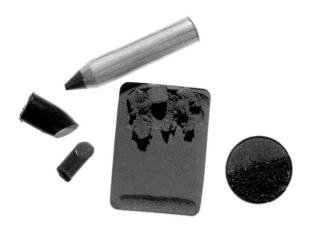

R E D H E A D

FAIR SKIN WAS ONCE THE HALLMARK OF GREAT BEAUTY
AND BREEDING. THOSE DAYS ARE GONE, THANK GOODNESS. VERY PALE
COMPLEXIONS ARE NOW SIMPLY AS LOVELY AS THE REST OF THE SPECTRUM OF SKIN
colors. Fair skin tends to be delicate and is often quite sensitive. The lack of melanin makes it
particularly susceptible to sun damage. It can be dry, and if you're a redhead it is often dusted
with freckles. Makeup should be sheer in texture and subtle in color, although strong eyes
or a deeply colored mouth can look all the more dramatic against such a pale backdrop.

HOW TO **FOUNDATION.** Freckled skin tends to be thin. Avoid heavy formulations, which mask freckles and lend an overall gray appearance. Instead, rejoice in your freckles. Tinted moisturizers even out skin tone, and sheer foundations will downplay freckles without hiding them. **CHEEKS.** Look for apri-cot blush tones or tawny, reddish browns for warmth. These shades will also blend in well with freckles. Pinks can be too cool and clash with red hair. **EYES.** Pale eyes look brighter under warm, brown tones. Copper and bronze undertones look particularly good when complementing red hair, which has an almost metal-lic quality. **LIPS.** Avoid strong pinks that will fight against the reddish undertone of the skin. Sheer lips or dark, brownish reds bring out the warmth of a fair complexion that may have hints of red, either due to natural coloring or sensi-tivity. Raisin colors and browns with orange undertones can look stunning on freckled skin.

BRUNETTE

UNDERNEATH HAIR THAT IS DARK BLONDE, CHESTNUT, OR INKY BLACK, your skin can be medium toned. You may have the sensitivities that plague lighter skin—except for a slightly higher tolerance to the sun—but your skin has a denser color that works very well with a range of different makeup looks. Medium-toned skin needs more color to liven up its yellower undertones. If your skin is on the sallow side, try colors with bluish hues, like plum browns and reds. Don't be afraid to wear dark, strong color on your lips or eyes. With your skin and hair, you can handle it. But remember: if you choose to lighten your hair color, you may need to adjust your makeup palette. Blonde hair, even with a medium complexion, requires a lighter touch and softer colors on the eyes and lips.

HOW TO

FOUNDATION AND POWDER. Bases with a lot of peach or pink in them will tend to make you look ruddy. Neutrals or even slightly yellow-toned foundations are better for evening out your complexion. Keep your powder light in texture and as close to the color of your foundation as possible. **LIPS.** You should normally avoid light lip color because it can make you look washed out. Experiment with a range of rich colors: plums, browns, reds, warm or muted mauvey pinks. If you like lighter lips, try these colors in a gloss. **EYES.** Dark eyes can carry more defined makeup, so look for dark, rich colors, like blacks or chocolate browns. Lighter eyes in a medium-toned face can handle drama well but may do better under more subtle washes of shadow. Often, whether you decide to keep your eyes soft or strong is a matter of your mood and the rest of your style. **CHEEKS.** A range of blushes is possible. For lighter medium tones, pale pinks and pinkish browns work well. Warmer colors, like dusty rose, will brighten darker skin.

1. Use a matte liquid foundation in a soft beige tone.

2. Dust with a light, translucent, banana-toned loose powder.

3. For warmth, apply a dusty-rose blush on the cheeks.

4. Define the eyes at the outer corners with a dark chocolate-brown powder liner at the base of the lashes.

5. For an eye with more depth, apply a deep hazel shadow to eyelids with a sponge-tip applicator.

6. To define eyes, apply black mascara.

7. Brighten the skin tone with a soft plum lipstick.

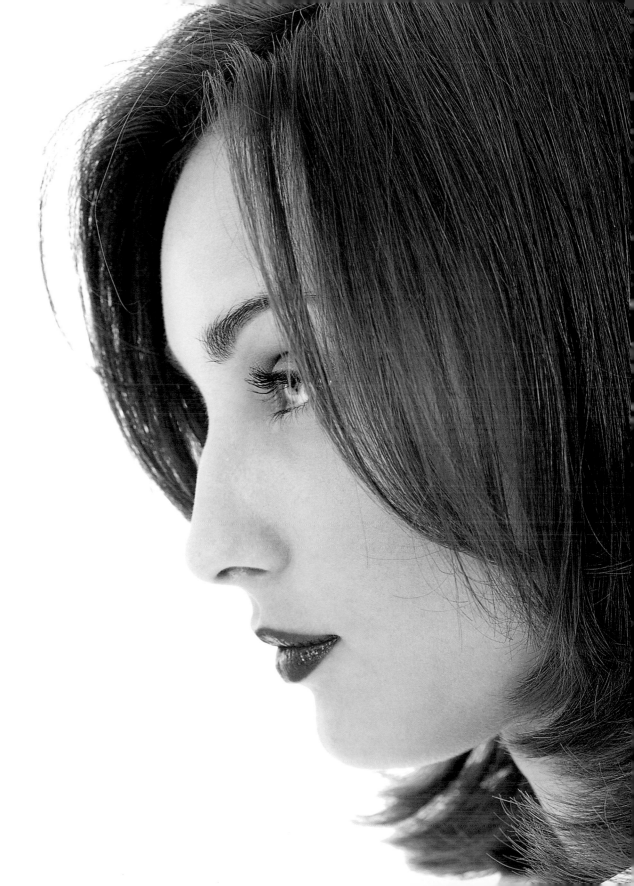

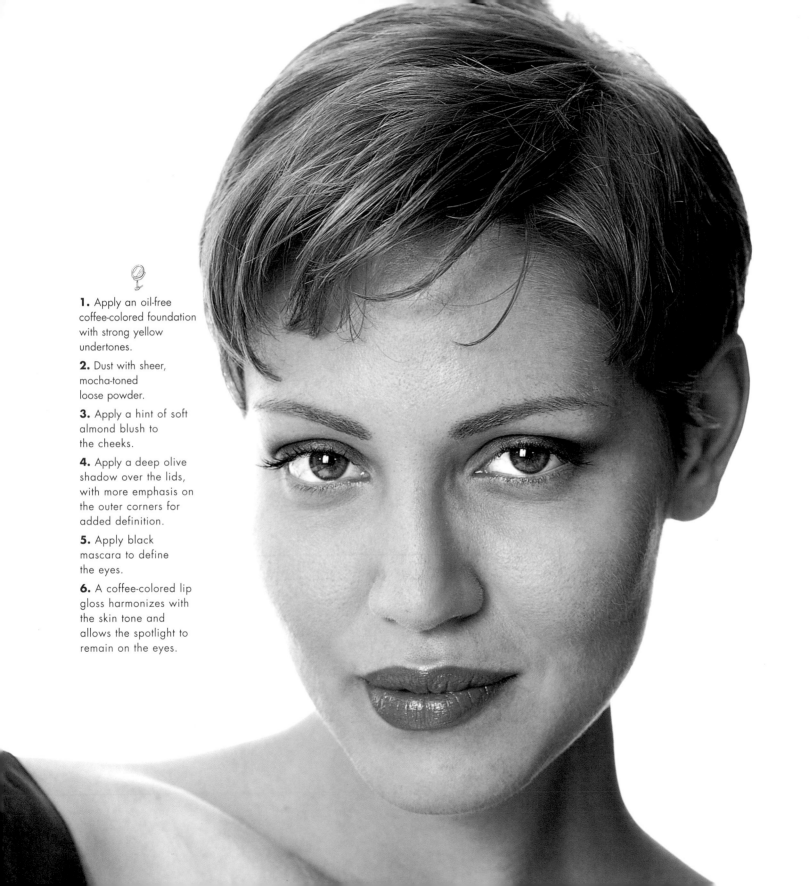

1. Apply an oil-free coffee-colored foundation with strong yellow undertones.

2. Dust with sheer, mocha-toned loose powder.

3. Apply a hint of soft almond blush to the cheeks.

4. Apply a deep olive shadow over the lids, with more emphasis on the outer corners for added definition.

5. Apply black mascara to define the eyes.

6. A coffee-colored lip gloss harmonizes with the skin tone and allows the spotlight to remain on the eyes.

D A R K

WOMEN WITH LIGHT-BROWN OR OLIVE-TONED SKIN ARE
DOUBLY BLESSED. BECAUSE THEIR FEATURES DON'T NEED AS MUCH
DEFINITION, THEY NEED LESS MAKEUP, BUT IF THEY WANT, THEY CAN WEAR MORE OF IT

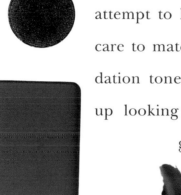

than women with lighter complexions. As a rule, darker complexions tend to be oilier, with slightly larger pores. They also do not wrinkle as easily, or react as sensitively to environmental factors like sun and cold. Darker skin—olive skin in particular—can have yellow undertones, which become muddy looking if too beige a foundation or powder is used in an attempt to lighten the skin. Take special care to match your powder to your foundation tone, or else your skin may wind up looking pasty. The basic rule is to go with your undertones, using them to complement the natural richness of your complexion.

FOUNDATION AND POWDER. As the skin gets darker, many brands of foundations, concealers, and powders come in increasingly orange tones. Avoid these. Look for rich-golden or deep-yellow undertones instead. **CHEEKS.** Warm coffee tones will shape your face without looking too dark. **EYES.** Colors can be strong and rich. Warm browns in chocolate, silver, bronze, or olive tones enhance the eyes without clashing with skin tone. Black mascara defines, even when you keep the rest of your makeup subtle. **LIPS.** Lipstick can be light or dramatic, as long as the color is a variation on a brown tone. Soft, velvety chocolate and red browns look natural, while plum and wine-colored browns, especially in a subtle gloss, will dress you up for evening. Pink tends to run too cool for such a warm skin tone, and orange does nothing. Avoid them both.

ASIAN

ASIAN SKIN TENDS TO BE VERY SMOOTH, ALMOST PORELESS, AND EVEN ON OLDER WOMEN, IT CAN LOOK YOUNG AND

fresh. Whether it's light, medium, or dark in color, it has yellow undertones, much like olive skin. Don't ignore them. You will end up looking ashen or chalky if you try to change the essential color of your skin with makeup. Stay away from pink and orange—they can look hard and garish—and avoid light brown, which will look muddy. Also steer clear of the chalky, white-toned powders designed to "lighten" Asian skin. They often lend a mask-like pallor and rob the skin of its natural warmth.

HOW TO **FOUNDATION AND POWDER.** Your complexion will look radiant and natural if you complement your skin tone with a base that has a little yellow in it. Powder should have a very fine, sheer texture and should not be too white. Match it to your foundation. **LIPS.** If your skin is pale, sheer pinks are lovely and soft. Stick with plum colors with brown, red, or mauve undertones. **EYES.** Narrow eyes need definition. Black eyeliner underneath and along the upper lid helps open up the eye area, as does softly smudged eyeshadow underneath and on the lid. Cool, dark grays work well for defining. Iridescents in sheer pale shades work beautifully on Asian eyes, adding light. Silver shadow brightens and adds luster to the eyes. If your eyebrows are thin, you may need to define and darken them with an eyebrow pencil, and if they are wiry, you can hold them in place with brow fix. Eyelashes that are straight and short can be curled with an eyelash curler for a more open look. **CHEEKS.** Soft, dusty pinks and plum colors lift a yellowish skin tone. To shape a round face, apply blush lower down on the apples of the cheeks, skirt the underside, then go higher and progressively narrower over the cheekbones.

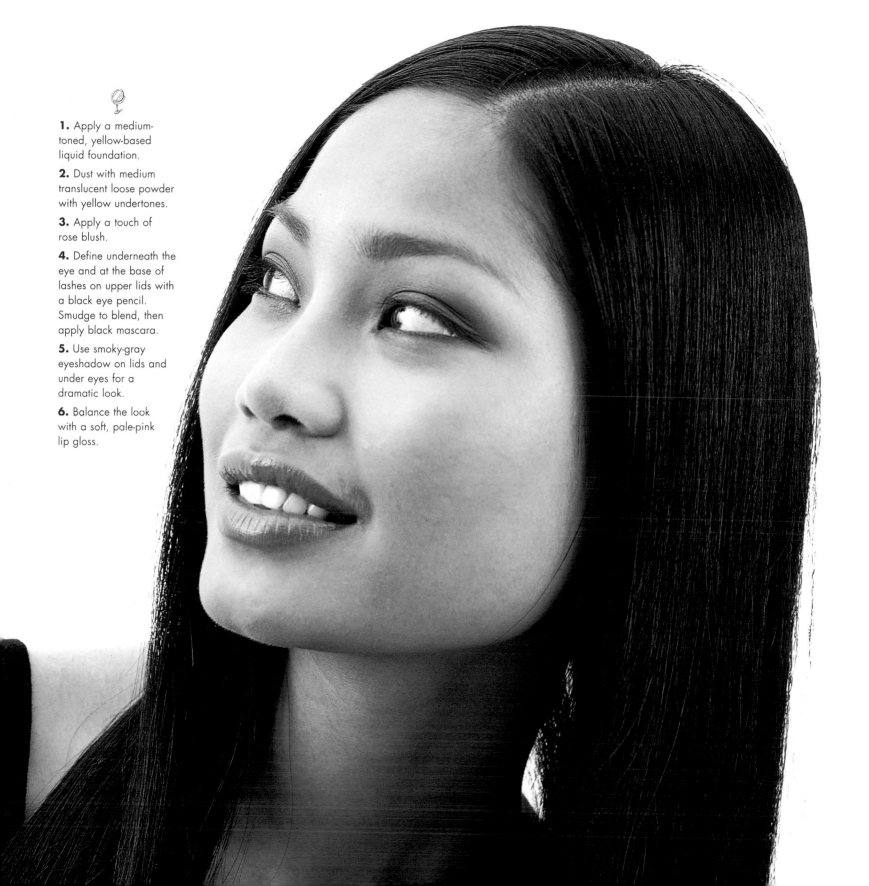

1. Apply a medium-toned, yellow-based liquid foundation.

2. Dust with medium translucent loose powder with yellow undertones.

3. Apply a touch of rose blush.

4. Define underneath the eye and at the base of lashes on upper lids with a black eye pencil. Smudge to blend, then apply black mascara.

5. Use smoky-gray eyeshadow on lids and under eyes for a dramatic look.

6. Balance the look with a soft, pale-pink lip gloss.

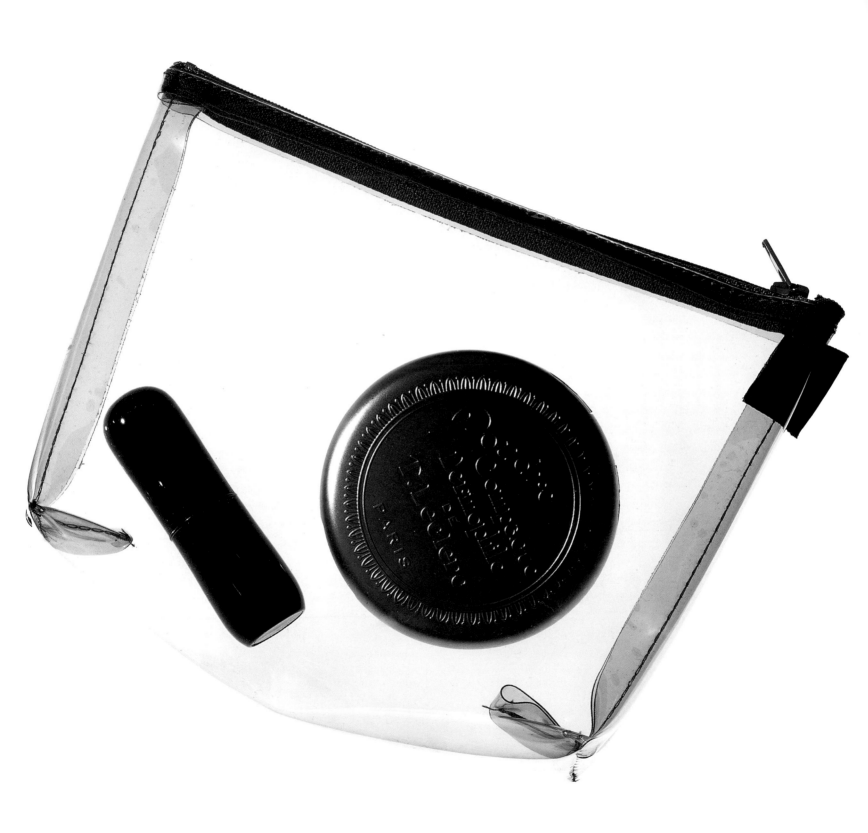

MAKEUP
WARDROBE

THE MINIMUM
- ☐ Lip balm

MINIMAL
- ☐ Lip balm
- ☐ Loose powder

MORE
- ☐ Lip balm
- ☐ Foundation
- ☐ Loose powder
- ☐ Mascara
- ☐ Brow definition, if necessary

FIVE-MINUTE MAKEUP
- ☐ Lip balm
- ☐ Foundation or concealer
- ☐ Loose powder
- ☐ Blush
- ☐ Soft liner
- ☐ Mascara
- ☐ Sheer lip color
- ☐ Brow definition, if necessary

FULL MAKEUP
- ☐ Lip balm
- ☐ Foundation
- ☐ Concealer, if necessary
- ☐ Powder
- ☐ Blush
- ☐ Brow definition, if necessary
- ☐ Eyeliner
- ☐ Eyeshadow
- ☐ Lip liner
- ☐ Lip color

ON TIRED DAYS OR BAD FACE DAYS
First try to revive yourself with a shower. Lie down and place cotton pads soaked with cold chamomile tea on your eyelids. Give yourself a revitalizing mask. Don't emphasize your eyes if you're tired. Use:
- a tinted moisturizer or foundation
- concealer, if necessary, but light enough to avoid emphasizing lines
- just enough blush to give you a healthy, just ran-around-the-block glow
- mascara to open up your eyes
- a light, neutral eyeshadow to even out skin tone on eyelids

EXERCISE CLASS
If you go to one of those classes where everyone is required not only to work out but to look fabulous while doing so, use
- water-resistant mascara
- gel blush, which works well on bare skin and is usually waterproof and long-lasting
- sheer lip color

BEACH OR POOL
Waterproof mascara, lip balm, and gloss, if you want. That's it.

WINTER
Skin usually loses its summer color, so adapt your foundation. Skin is also drier in winter. Use more of a richer moisturizer, or switch to a moisturizing foundation. Stronger lip colors look good in winter.

WEDDING
You'll want a professional to handle your makeup on this special day. Or go to a professional a few weeks before your date and learn how to apply the look you want. You can find a makeup artist through bridal or beauty magazines.

PARTY
Although parties provide an opportunity to experiment with makeup, make sure you feel comfortable with what you're wearing. You want to put on your makeup and forget about it, especially if you're dancing all night. Long-lasting makeup helps. A look with simple eyes and strong lips works well.

TRAVEL
- Airplane cabins have next to zero humidity, so bring lip balm, moisturizer, and even water to spritz your face.
- Don't wear foundation while you're flying—it will dry your skin. Instead, emphasize your eyes or lips.
- On the run? Keep lip color, lip balm, and powder in your purse.
- Pack makeup in travel-sized containers.

PUBLIC SPEAKING
Define your basic makeup a little more, and use more powder, especially if there are going to be lights shining on you.

INTERVIEWS
Simple, polished, and not overly made-up. Avoid really strong colors.

CASUAL WORKDAYS
Casual workdays do not mean no makeup. You still need to look pulled together and professional. The casual factor may simply mean skipping foundation and using powder, a neutral eyeshadow, mascara, blush, and lip gloss.

Survival Gear

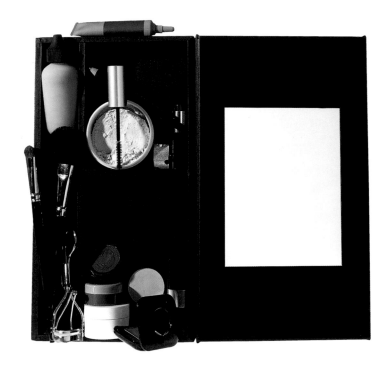

DAILY
Skin-care wardrobe:
☐ Makeup remover
☐ Face cleanser
☐ Moisturizer
☐ Sunblock
☐ Astringent or toner
(optional)

Skin-care tools:
☐ Cotton pads
☐ Sea sponge
☐ Washcloth

Makeup wardrobe:
☐ Foundation
☐ Loose powder
☐ Concealer
☐ Brow pencil
☐ Eyeliner
☐ Eyeshadow
☐ Mascara
☐ Blush
☐ Lip color
☐ Lip pencil

Makeup tools:
☐ Latex wedges
☐ Small sea sponge
☐ Cotton swabs
☐ Tweezers
☐ Eyelash curler
☐ Eye-pencil sharpener

Makeup brushes:
☐ Loose powder
☐ Blush
☐ Eyeshadow
☐ Brow
☐ Lip
☐ Eyeliner

Morning and night:
☐ Moisturizer on face and neck
☐ Eye cream
☐ Lip balm

Emergencies:
☐ Spot lotion for pimples

ONCE A WEEK
(minimum):
☐ Exfoliant

ONCE A MONTH
(minimum):
☐ Facial mask

first aid.

The hard part: there are thousands of makeup products, hundreds of cleansing regimens, countless opportunities to experiment. The easy part: there's only one you. The following pages will help you adapt to whatever environment you're thrown into, from counter to podium, with ways to maintain your face so you won't have to save face.

Emergency Fix-Ups

Sometimes when you're applying makeup, a small goof can escalate into a big mess if you're not sure how to correct it. The cardinal fix tip is to stay calm. After that, here are a few more that may help.

FOUNDATION. If you've applied too much foundation and don't have time to start over, go over your face with a damp sea sponge, blending downward and out. You'll thin the base and remove the excess foundation. • If you have patches of dry skin on your face and your foundation seems to cling there, moisturize the dry spots before applying a silicone-based foundation, which clings less and covers more smoothly. Use a damp sea sponge to blend.

EYES. If you blink a little mascara onto your cheek, you can whisk the smudge off with a cotton swab dipped in eye-makeup remover. • To prevent your eyeliner from smudging underneath your eye, dip a cotton swab in a little loose powder and smooth it over your eyeliner. This will set the pencil. • To help prevent your eyeliner from creasing, apply a bit of loose powder to your lids with a latex wedge before you use your eye pencil. Priming your eyelids with powder provides a clean, dry base for your eyeliner and helps it last longer.

LIPS. To ensure that your lipstick lasts, blot your lips after applying it, then reapply and blot again. Two layers, with the excess blotted off, will hold the color better. • If your lipstick bleeds around the edges, avoid gloss formulations (matte and cream have more staying power). Powder around the outline of your lips, and use a lip pencil to help prevent bleeding. • To keep lipstick off your front teeth, an old trick is to insert your index finger into your mouth, then press your lips together and pull the finger out. The excess lipstick will cling to your finger, not your teeth.

Cleaning Up

REMOVING MAKEUP FROM YOUR FACE. Some makeup artists say that the best, gentlest way to remove makeup—including gloss, pencil, and lipstick—is simply with moisturizer and tissues or flat cotton pads. • Liquid and gel-type makeup removers are less likely to irritate your eyes than oil-based products. And since they are more easily absorbed by the skin, they're less likely to cause those little bumps under your eyes. • Wayward fibers from cotton balls may irritate your eyes, so use pads with a lower shed factor. And if you wear contact lenses, always take them out before removing your eye makeup.

REMOVING MAKEUP FROM YOUR CLOTHES. Lipstick, especially, has a nagging tendency to come off your lips when you don't want it to. If any makeup item is rubbing off too easily, it may be because it's too thick (culprits: a product that's oil-based or past its prime, or a moisturizer underneath that's too oily). • Use powder to hold down wetter products that you suspect might rub off. • One effective tool is hair spray. Spray the spot immediately, then blot. Lipstick can also be removed with a non-oil-based makeup remover, a non-gel toothpaste, dry-cleaning solvent, or a piece of soft white bread. After applying any of these techniques, wash the garment as usual. If color remains, try soaking in water and ammonia. • Also, don't forget the handy dinner-party, wine-on-the-tablecloth system of stain removal: a dab of club soda, then salt. • If all else fails, take it to the dry cleaner and explain both what the stain consists of and what you've done to try to salvage the situation.

CLEANING MAKEUP BRUSHES. Strong detergents, even the ones actually packaged to clean brushes, can dry out bristles. It's better for your brushes if you use warm water and a mild soap or shampoo. Wash them as you'd wash your hair. Place a small amount of shampoo in the palm of your hand, then add some water and rinse the brushes until they're clean. Gently pat dry, repoint the tips, and let them dry overnight. Caution: never soak brushes overnight, since the glue could start dissolving and cause the bristles to fall out. As an alternative, you can use a dry-cleaning solution for makeup brushes. Apply solution to a tissue and wipe the brush (not against the grain) until the tissue comes out clean.

Buying Cosmetics

AT THE COSMETICS COUNTER. Know what you're shopping for, and make your personal priorities known. Keep a shopping list in the bathroom, the way you keep a grocery list in the kitchen. • There is no need to buy an entire line of cosmetics. You may like various products from different lines. • Know your skin type. • Ask for free samples and take as many as you can carry. Product literature can't hurt, either. • Be wary of cosmetic-counter lighting. If possible, go outside the store to see what a cosmetic looks like in natural daylight. • Reveal your budget. • Ask questions. Don't buy anything you're uncertain about. If you do wind up buying something that you later find you don't care for, remember that most major companies have return policies for unopened products, and often for opened ones, too. • Gauge your mood before you go shopping. If you go on a spree when you're feeling depressed or unattractive, you'll look at your purchases a few days later and wonder what you were thinking. Try going to a movie instead. • If you have a favorite makeup product that the manufacturer has discontinued, you might be able to get it custom blended at some salons. • Don't test foundation or other makeup on the back of your hand: your skin there is a different shade than on your face. Place it at your jawline. If it disappears into your skin, it's the right color. • Makeup brushes made of natural fibers are better than synthetic ones because natural bristles are softer. They're also more expensive. Art supply stores can be a great place to buy brushes if you know what you're looking for. They're often less expensive than brushes made specifically for makeup. Brushes can last a long time if you care for them properly. • You can also save a lot of money by buying some types of makeup at the drugstore. If you know the color that's best for you, you can buy lipsticks there; you can at least purchase all your mascaras, eyeliners, and lip liners at the drugstore. The one item that's important to purchase at a makeup counter is foundation—it's the only way you can be sure you have the right color. • And if you've bought the makeup but don't think you're putting it to its best use, you can always spend a bit more for makeup lessons from a freelance makeup artist or local cosmetics store.

THE SHELF LIFE OF MAKEUP.

Most manufacturers of cosmetics don't do you the favor of providing expiration dates. Some items, like lipstick and eye pencils, can last indefinitely, though you should always be on the lookout for uncharacteristic smells or consistencies. Other products, like mascara, eyeliner, and face powder, need to be replaced frequently, not only because they're subject to germ accumulation, but because you use them in areas that are easily infected. The life span of your cosmetics also varies depending on where you store them. Though it may be convenient, the bathroom is one of the worst places to keep makeup. The room's humidity can melt lipsticks and cause foundation to clump. Here are general guidelines for shelf life after you've opened the containers. **Sunscreen:** Two years. After that—less if it's been stored in a high-heat area—sunscreen begins to lose its effectiveness. There's usually an expiration date somewhere on the container. **Eye and lip pencils:** Three years, possibly longer. If you're suspicious, sharpen the suspect end away.

Eyeshadow, blush, gloss: Two years. **Foundation and moisturizer:** One year. Keeping it in the fridge helps sustain its life and makes for an invigorating skin-care regimen. Apply it with a foundation brush to avoid the germs your fingers can bring. **Eyeliner:** Six months. **Face powder:** Six months. Since dampness is face powder's mortal enemy, don't store it in the bathroom. And when you're applying it, try sprinkling some powder onto a clean surface and dipping the brush in this, instead of dipping the brush into the container. **Mascara:** Three months. Never share your mascara or use saliva to thin it or point the brush. **Eye cream:** Three to six months. Because it's designed to moisturize the sensitive area around your eyes, eye cream is often manufactured with few or no preservatives, which means that its shelf life is more limited. Again, refrigerating helps. **Bleach:** Bleach for upper lips has an expiration date that shouldn't be ignored. When the ingredients age and separate, they not only lose their ability to bleach effectively, they actually start acting as a dye and may leave you with an orange mustache.

How to Read a Label

NATURAL INGREDIENTS. The word "natural" can be bent a long way under current FDA guidelines, so if you want a true alternative to blockbuster cosmetic products, look for labels that say "chemical free." For one thing, that could mean flower-derived pigments instead of the coal tar that most big companies use to color their lipsticks. But it also means a narrower range of color choices and less staying power than the processed versions. And anyway, technically, coal tar is natural, too.

ESSENTIAL OILS.

Essential oils, like jasmine, rose, chamomile, and lemon, are available in little vials at specialty stores and can be used

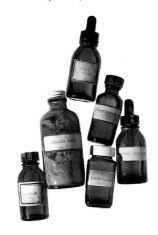

in a wide variety of homemade cosmetics, which adherents say are fresher, safer, more fun, and sometimes more economical than the big-brand ones. They're superpotent: 6,000 pounds of jasmine, for instance, yields 1 gallon of oil (for external use only). Mix one to five drops of essential oil with a quart of spring water to make a cleanser, toner, and compress. Lemon, lavender, and geranium oils are particularly effective against oily skin, and rose oil fights dry skin—though FDA regulations prevent manufacturers of these oils from making any health-based claims for them.

"What I needed to do in beauty was to come up with a New York formula. You know, protect your face against the pollution, the dirt, the sun—everything seems to be at a higher velocity here in New York."

DONNA KARAN

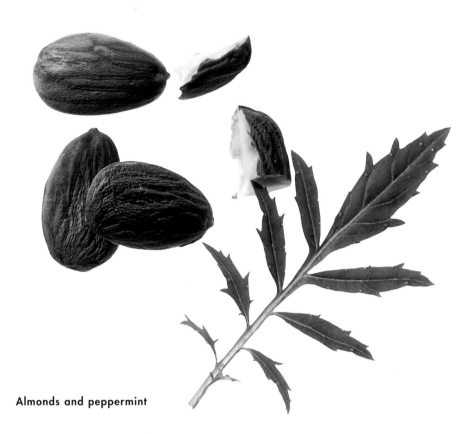

Almonds and peppermint

Skin Talk

ALCOHOL, SD ALCOHOL 10-40: Alcohol is frequently the base of astringents and toners. Though it has strong cleansing properties, it can dry out the skin.

ALLANTOIN: A skin-soothing ingredient often found in moisturizers, lotions, and gels.

ALMONDS: Almond oil and extract are effective moisturizers; finely crushed almonds are often used as an exfoliant in creams.

ALOE: An anti-inflammatory ingredient found in many lotions and creams. It also helps heal wounds.

ANTIOXIDANTS: Vitamins—mainly betacarotene, vitamin A, and vitamin E—that counter the damaging effects of free radicals.

AROMATHERAPY: The use of certain scents to produce sensations of relaxation, coolness, and refreshment, aromatherapy is now also used in electrolysis sessions to make the experience easier. **Invigorating scents** include clove, rosemary, spruce, juniper, lemon, and peppermint. **Stress relievers** include vanilla, nutmeg, and orange. **Relaxants** include jasmine, chamomile, marjoram, lavender, and rose. **Aphrodisiacs** include sandalwood, ylang-ylang, and sage.

BEESWAX: A common ingredient in creams and balms, beeswax can soothe and condition chapped lips; honey also has healing properties and is a natural humectant.

COLLAGEN AND ELASTIN: Two layers of the skin that hold water. The external application of collagen or elastin has not been found to be effective, though collagen injections can cause temporary skin-plumping and fill in wrinkles.

CUCUMBER: Containing vitamins A and C, and a large proportion of water, cucumber is an effective soother of skin inflammations; it also reduces enlarged pores and helps control oiliness.

DERMIS: The second, thicker layer of the skin, under the epidermis.

EMOLLIENT: An ingredient in a lotion or moisturizer intended to soften the skin.

EPIDERMIS: The thin, outermost layer of the skin.

ESSENTIAL OILS: Highly concentrated oils derived from any of a variety of plants and used in natural beauty products and perfumes. Each type of oil is thought to have a specific therapeutic effect.

FREE RADICALS: The "rust" of the body, free radicals are oxidants generated by sunlight and pollutants (especially smoking); they damage the skin by destabilizing its natural oxygen and weakening cells.

GLYCERIN: A common ingredient in moisturizers and makeup, glycerin helps keep skin hydrated.

HUMECTANT: In a face cream or lotion, an ingredient that triggers skin cells to retain moisture.

HYALURONIC ACID: A common ingredient in moisturizers (and in the lower layers of your skin), hyaluronic acid is an effective humectant.

LANOLIN: Effective at keeping the skin supple, but causes irritation in some.

LIPIDS: Structural matter in cells made of fats and water, lipids keep your cells from dehydrating. Some moisturizers contain manmade lipids known as ceramides.

MAXIMUM COVER: The most coverage a foundation can give: opaque, and good for camouflaging minor blemishes.

MINERAL OIL: Found in a vast array of cosmetics, mineral oil is the carrier of active ingredients and is a mildly effective humectant itself. It is popular because it doesn't irritate.

NONCOMEDOGENIC: A product that is less likely to clog your pores.

OCCLUSIVE INGREDIENTS: Ingredients that help the skin absorb and retain moisture.

OIL: Oils—both natural and chemical—keep skin moisturized internally. Oil-based moisturizers are good for dry skin; makeup removers are generally oil based.

PABA: Para-aminobenzoic acid, a chemical sunscreen that works by absorbing ultraviolet light (thus shielding your skin from it); causes allergic reactions in some cases.

PANTHENOL: A commonly used skin soother.

PARABENS: A class of preservatives frequently used in cosmetics, less likely to cause allergic reactions than their harsher ancestors. The most common are methylparaben, propylparaben, and butylparaben.

PEPPERMINT: Cooling and soothing in lotions and night creams, peppermint can also be boiled into a moisturizing tea.

PETROLATUM: A common moisturizing ingredient with a strong record for delivering moisture to the skin and not causing irritation.

PORES: Openings for sebaceous glands on the skin's surface. Their size is inherited. Larger pores usually have more active oil glands.

SALICYLIC ACID: Used frequently in acne preparations for its ability to exfoliate the skin, but can be irritating.

SEBACEOUS GLANDS: Glands throughout the body responsible for secreting oils. Contrary to legend, the sebaceous glands on the face operate independently of diet. They'll generate the same amount of oil whether or not you eat that pizza. And if you overscrub your face, your sebaceous glands will produce more oil.

SEBUM: An oily, fatty substance secreted by the sebaceous glands. Impacted pores are usually caused by sebum build-up.

TEA-TREE OIL: A plant extract that can be used against acne, bad breath, and even dandruff. The FDA, however, does not allow manufacturers of tea-tree oil to make claims for their product's efficacy.

THALASSOTHERAPY: Literally "seaweed treatment," this is a spa-administered pampering, using seaweed-derived gels to nourish and moisturize the skin.

TONER: Often alcohol-based, toner can reduce the production of sebum by as much as 15 percent.

WATER: Steady intake of water—eight cups a day —is absolutely crucial to maintaining good skin and general well-being. It's what we're mostly made of, after all.

WITCH HAZEL: A mild astringent containing oils from the leaves and bark of the witch hazel shrub; safe for many sensitive complexions, though bear in mind that witch hazel does contain alcohol, despite some labels that say it doesn't.

YOGURT: An effective topical treatment medium for oily and combination skin.

ZINC OXIDE: Opaque "nonchemical" sunscreen that, unlike PABA (which is more effective), works by reflecting ultraviolet light. It and its cousin, titanium dioxide, are most often used in SPF-formula makeup.

Vitamins

THE FREE RADICAL/ANTIOXIDANT THEORY. Peel an apple and watch it brown. That, scientists speculate, is what happens in the human aging process. Like the apple flesh exposed to air, human flesh is oxidizing. Sun exposure and pollutants generate oxidants known as **free radicals**— destructive molecules in the body that cause cell damage by stealing electrons from other body cells, destabilizing oxygen molecules, and weakening or killing cells in the process. In other words, free radicals are the rust of your body. While the antioxidant theory is still in its infancy, we do know for sure that sunlight and smoking are The Enemy. There is hope, however. Our bodies contain natural **antioxidants** that combine with free radicals, preventing them from damaging DNA and enzymes in the skin. The big three antioxidants are **betacarotene, vitamin A,** and **vitamin E.** They can be taken in supplements or eaten in green vegetables like spinach and broccoli.

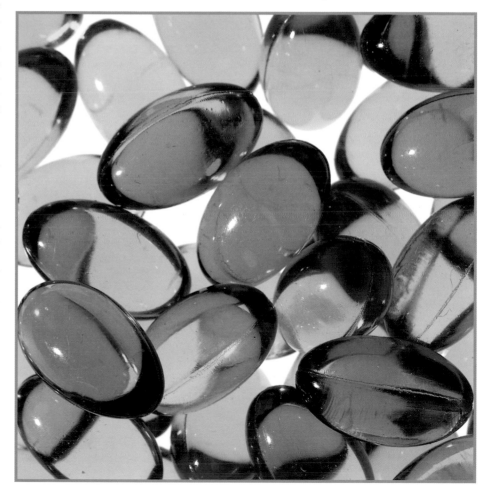

VITAMIN LEXICON. The skin is the first organ of the body to reflect deficiencies and excesses of vitamins and minerals. Fortunately, skin diseases caused by inadequate nutrition are uncommon today. In fact, often it's vitamin overdoses that cause more trouble than, say, scurvy, as any carrot-juice addict with a faint orange glow can attest. **Water-soluble vitamins** include vitamin C and the B-complex vitamins, meaning they're not stored in your fat cells, so it's important to have a steady intake of them. **Fat-soluble vitamins** include vitamins A, D, E, and K. They can be ingested with less frequency, since your body is capable of storing them.

VITAMIN A: Present in green vegetables, carrots, and liver products, vitamin A helps keep skin elastic and supple; it also fights dryness. Symptoms of vitamin A deficiency are the same as those of excess: the skin begins to peel, follicles loosen, and hair loss may occur.

VITAMIN B_3 (NIACIN): A steady intake of niacin, which is plentiful in meat and grains, contributes to a healthy, glowing complexion. Deficiency can result in a skin rash called pellagra.

VITAMIN B_{12}: Since vitamin B_{12} has long been used to counter anemia, B_{12} deficiency and anemia symptoms (paleness, lack of energy, swollen tongue) tend to overlap. B_{12} "shots" have had their periods in vogue but haven't been proven to do much—unless, of course, you're anemic.

VITAMIN C: An important antioxidant (think lemon juice on cut apples) that helps maintain blood vessels, elastin fibers, and collagen. Deficiency results in the infamous scurvy, characterized by bleeding under the skin and in the gums. Megadoses of C may cause diarrhea and, because it's an acid, kidney stones in some cases.

VITAMIN D: The skin actually serves vitamin D, and not the reverse, processing sunlight to produce this valuable energy source (hence the feelings of lethargy in northern winters, when sunlight and vitamin D are at low points). Vitamin D also guards against bone disease.

VITAMIN E: Vitamin E is considered an antioxidant and is a popular external remedy for skin damage, but not all the claims made on its behalf have been substantiated. We do know that it helps transport nutrients to skin cells; too much E, however, can block the reception of other fat-soluble vitamins, like A and D.

VITAMIN K: Present in leafy green vegetables and manufactured by bacteria in the intestine, vitamin K is key to promoting blood clotting.

The Seasons

When you find a makeup look you like, it's not necessary to change it entirely each season, yet adjustments may be necessary if your skin is paler in the dead of winter than in the middle of summer. With the change in season, you may also be in the mood for a change in lipstick color or texture. It's a quick and inexpensive way to adapt your makeup wardrobe. Also, your skin care regimen may need to adapt to the changing climate.

WINTER: Among other things, winter means a battle against dry skin. Cracked skin is an open invitation to infection or an acne breakout. To avoid patchy dry spots on your face, use a light moisturizer in layers: apply it thinly to your face, wait for it to dry, then apply another layer. Or use a heavier, non-water-based moisturizer. • Use mild cleansers and indulge in a nourishing mask every so often. Apply lip balm several times daily to avoid chapping. • Hot showers may feel good, but they're hard on fragile winter skin. Try lowering the temperature and time. • For the same reasons, a long post-workout sauna session can stress your skin as well. • Wearing a scarf helps in the fight against windburn and those tiny broken blood vessels on the nose and cheeks (which can be caused by sudden changes in temperature, among other things). • Most women's skin is paler than usual in the winter. You might need a lighter-colored foundation until the sun makes its return. • Reduce paleness with rosy blush hues. Add depth around the eyes with deeper shadows, and find a good moisturizing lipstick.

SPRING: Spring is a good time to get a professional facial, to shed your winter skin and prepare for warmer weather. It's also a good time to see a makeup consultant to learn about new textures and colors, and lighter makeup for the summer ahead. • As it gets warmer outside, pay special attention to where you store your makeup. Try keeping your lipsticks and pencils in the fridge. They won't melt, and you'll even be able to apply them with more precision. • Powder helps hold makeup in place on rainy days. Color your lips with lip pencil, then lipstick, and then add a thin layer of powder. Or draw a fine line of eyeliner near your lashes—to create bounds for your eyeshadow—then powder.

SUMMER: The sun. Though sun-derived skin damage is a year-round issue, summer means being especially careful in the sun. A disheartening statistic: there are more than 800,000 new cases of skin cancer diagnosed in the United States every year. • Avoid exposure between ten in the morning and four in the afternoon, when the sun is most intense. If you're going to be outdoors between those

"In the factory we make cosmetics. In the store we sell hope."

CHARLES REVSON

hours, wear sunscreen and protective clothing. • Makeup without an SPF rating is at least a physical block against harmful ultraviolet radiation. (SPF means sun-protection factor; if you wear a sunblock with an SPF of 8, you have eight times more protection from the sun than you'd have if you weren't wearing any sunblock at all.) Still, if you know you're going to be outside, you must wear a sunscreen with your makeup. • SPF 15 sunblock is sufficient for pretty much everybody, as long as you use enough of it. Translation: use a lot. Too-thin coverage won't help you at all. • SPF formulas are not cumulative: if you use a moisturizer with SPF 8 and a sunblock with SPF 4, your protection is still 8, not 12. • Gel sunblocks are better than creams for oily skin. • If you've just waxed or shaved, don't expose your smooth, sensitive skin to the sun. You could get a rash. **Makeup formulas.** Opinion is divided on the virtues of makeup and foundations with built-in sunscreens. They're easy to use, and they're better than nothing, but they're generally heavier and oilier than the regular versions. Many dermatologists recommend wearing a sunscreen under makeup instead, to provide more even sun protection. If you can, let the sunscreen soak in for at least ten minutes before applying your makeup. **Swimming.** Never wear a sunscreen labeled "reapply after swimming" if you are swimming. It won't protect you in the water. • Be sure to dry your face with a clean towel after you've been swimming: you'll wipe away salt and chlorine residue that could dry your skin later. Then reapply sunscreen. • Another famous summer concern is mosquitoes. Serendipitously, some skin care products, like Avon's Skin-So-Soft moisturizer, keep the bugs away and smell good in the process. **Faking it.** There's always the sun-free tanning scene. Recently introduced products include a lotion that stimulates melanin production, rather than suntan-shaded dyes. The product has been tested on pigs, who maintained a healthy bronze glow for four months. • And speaking of dyes, if you're considering getting your eyelashes dyed for the summer, bear in mind that the FDA has not approved the coal-tar-based dye that most salons use—and it

hasn't approved henna, either. Both can cause allergic reactions.

FALL: Like spring, fall is an ideal time to visit a facialist. Buckle down for colder weather, but fall's climate can be unpredictable. It's a good idea to be prepared for too much sun, too much cold, too much wind, or all of the above. That means sunscreen and lip balm, as usual. You may also want to consider adjusting your makeup palette to complement your fall wardrobe.

Taking It on the Road

PACKING. Pack your makeup in smaller containers (loose powder can be put in a little plastic box with a sifter top), available in makeup supply stores. Even lipsticks can be cut and mashed into a mini lip-palette box—a vitamin box from the drugstore works well. Don't take a lot of brushes on a vacation. The most you'll need will be a powder brush, a blush brush, a sponge-tip applicator, and a retractable lip brush. Think about the purpose of your trip. Business or pleasure? For a business trip, you'll

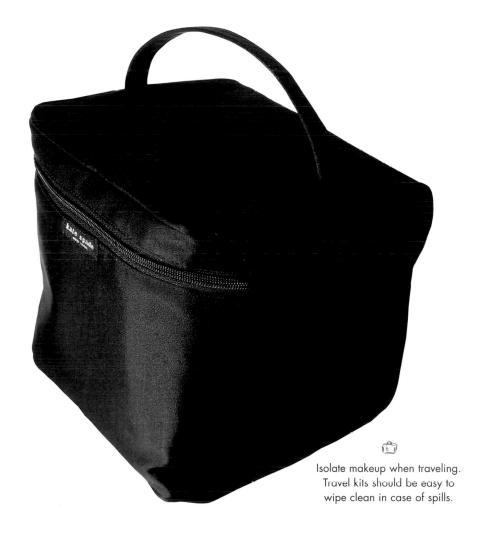

Isolate makeup when traveling. Travel kits should be easy to wipe clean in case of spills.

pretty much need what you use every day at home. If you're going to be vacationing somewhere warm, you'll need to think about your makeup a little differently. You'll probably get some color on your face, so you might even want to leave your regular foundation behind—and you'll need sunscreen, of course. Sheer face tints and moisturizers work well in warmer climates, and powder can help minimize shine and create a polished evening look. Keep your eye makeup simple. One eyeshadow and/or one shimmery highlighter, a powder-based eye pencil (they hold up better in the heat), and mascara are all you might need. For lips, decide on no more than three colors. Lip balm is crucial, not just for the health of your lips, but for toning down your lipsticks as your face takes on color. And take concealer, in case of a breakout. To keep cosmetics from melting when traveling, keep the following in mind: Refrigerate them in the summer months so that they're not already soft before you head out. Never leave them in a glove compartment or locker. When picnicking in the sun, place them in the cooler along with your drinks.

WHILE YOU'RE TRAVELING.

The super-dry pressurized air in an airplane cabin can wreak havoc on your skin. In general, avoid wearing foundations and blushes on the plane: they may make your face look puffy. Eye makeup is fine, or bring an eyelash curler. Use plenty of lip balm, either by itself or under your lipstick. Apply extra moisturizer if your flight is more than a couple of hours long. Also, drink plenty of water, especially if you're having drinks onboard.

UPON ARRIVAL: GLOBAL MAKEUP

LONDON. Though young Londoners are famous for trend-spotting and an intense fashion consciousness, in general British women wear less makeup than women in comparable urban centers. Some people say that British skin looks healthier than the average, perhaps because of continual exposure to moisturizing air and all that milk and cream. Most English women wouldn't dream of covering their rosy

skin with face paint (how soon we forgot the impact of Mary Quant cosmetics). And then there's also a tacit understanding that low-maintenance makeup is best—it just doesn't do to look as though one is a slave to glamour, and great skin is favored over a great makeup job.

NEW YORK. The career woman meets the time crunch, and the result is a full-makeup look, but one that can be applied in record time—in the back of a taxicab, if necessary. New York women purchase more makeup than women in most European cities. When they're wearing makeup, they're striving for a strong, professional look, and a "natural" look usually means concealer, light foundation, and mascara, if that.

PARIS. Perception isn't a far cry from reality in the world capital of beauty. French women opt most often for simple but assertive makeup. The red-lipstick-and-black-eyeliner look is far from uncommon. And, of course, in the culture that invented the word "salon" (not to mention "chic"), *Parisiennes* pride themselves on being *au courant* about the last word in skin care. Possibly in the interest of nipping eye wrinkles in the bud, smiling is frowned upon.

ROME. In the Italian capital, less makeup is more, but because of suntans and predominantly darker and olive complexions, makeup shades differ from those found in more northern climates. The emphasis is on lipstick first, then perhaps some eyeliner. But understatement is the boldest statement of all.

TOKYO. More than twice as many skin-care products as makeup products are purchased in Tokyo; in the United States that proportion is reversed. The perception is that Japanese women spend more time making themselves up than women in other places, and it is true that foundation tends to be considered more a staple than an option in Tokyo. Also popular are skin-whitening creams that claim to create a more "balanced" complexion (in our opinion, these creams tend to sabotage a naturally beautiful skin color). Japanese women are also much

more interested in experimenting with lip color than with eye makeup.

Occasions

INTERVIEWS. Your goal here is to look serious and professional—and, of course, to get the job. Interview makeup should be subtle (you don't want them to think you obsess over your looks) and consistent with what you're wearing. • Draw the interviewer's attention to your eyes with mascara and possibly a soft brown eyeliner. Don't wear lipstick that's too bright or glossy. You want the interviewer to pay attention to your brilliant answers rather than be distracted by your mouth. • As with any adrenaline-producing situation, you may perspire more than usual during or in anticipation of an interview. Powder is important, and bring some along with you in case you need to refresh beforehand.

PUBLIC SPEAKING. Making yourself up for a speech depends on how far you'll be from your audience and what type of lighting will be used. If lights are intense, you might want to apply a little extra powder to avoid shine. • Don't overdo your makeup, or your audience will pay more attention to it than to your speech. Use your regular regimen, with a little added definition around the eyes and lips.

TELEVISION. MAKEUP. Television programs almost always have a makeup artist who knows the show's particular lighting and camera quirks, so if you're making an appearance, inquire beforehand so you can rest easy as long as you're scrubbed and arrive early enough. • You'll be wearing more makeup than you're used to: yellow-toned foundation, concealer, a lot of powder, somewhat brighter or deeper lip color and blush, and more defined eye makeup. TV makeup artists use matte textures almost exclusively because glossier finishes can be distracting under bright lights. If you're on your own, get a lesson from a makeup artist with television experience or follow full makeup guidelines and keep powder on hand. Under hot lights, your face will tend to get shiny. **CLOTHES.** Wear comfortable clothes in safe colors: neutrals like navy and beige look good on television. Dark colors are slimming. Black can give definition if there is shape to the garment, or it can be accented with a bright-colored blouse or scarf. White is too bright for television. Blues, dusty pink, magenta, and deep reds all show well on TV. Bright red may cause some dissolution in a garment's silhouette. Don't wear noisy jewelry. Make sure arms and legs aren't bare; they may appear shiny. **HAIR.** Hair looks best off the face. Bangs may make you look young, but they can undermine your authority. If you have a tendency to toy with your hair, pull it back. • The camera can add weight to your face, so accent your best attributes.

Troubleshooting Face Problems

SKIN

Ashy skin. Ashy skin or patches of light skin are particularly conspicuous in darker complexions. It occurs when precocious skin cells make their way to the epidermis before they've developed sufficient pigment. A moisturizer with a mild concentration of alpha-hydroxy acids, and perhaps a weekly regimen of sloughing cream, should take care of the problem.

Facial hair. The amount of facial hair is genetically determined, but it will fluctuate with changing hormone levels. Consequently, the Pill can cause an increase in facial-hair growth. Also, older women tend to become hairier as the level of estrogen in the body falls relative to testosterone. The easiest way to treat upper-lip hair at home is bleaching. Be sure to follow the package instructions carefully—leaving the cream on too long could cause irritation. Also, don't use bleaching products that have expired. They won't bleach your upper-lip hair, but they may make it turn orange. Bleaching, however, is not a good idea if your skin is dark. Chemical cream depilatories dissolve hair at the root but need to be used quite frequently and may irritate the

skin. Waxing—applying strips of wax to the hairy area and then ripping it off—works wonderfully, removing hair at the root. You should go to a professional, though, and be aware that waxing can cause sensitive skin to break out. Electrolysis, the destruction of hair follicles by running a mild electric current through them, is the only permanent method of hair removal. It can be pricey and often has to be repeated several times. Shaving is the one bad solution for facial hair. It does not make hair grow back faster or thicker, as reputed, but it may irritate the skin.

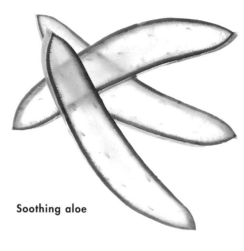

Soothing aloe

Plus, stubble on a woman is unlikely to have the same turn-on quotient as stubble on Bruce Willis.

Nose hairs. They're extremely important for keeping bits of dust and other foreign matter out of the sinus cavities; on the other hand, they should be kept in the nose, where they belong. Nose hairs on both men and women often grow longer with age. Trim them with tiny clippers created especially for the purpose.

Pimples. Unfortunately, acne does not cease to exist after puberty. When breakouts are frequent, consult a dermatologist. The cardinal rule is to avoid touching your face with your hands. Most other cases of adult acne are brought about by stress and hormonal fluctuations. It can usually be treated with an over-the-

counter benzoyl-peroxide cream; if that's not cutting it, you can also use prescriptive drugs like Retin-A, AHAs, Accutane (pretty strong stuff), and even the Pill. For occasional blemishes, stick to your cleansing routine, and eventually they should clear up. • Alcohol-based astringents will dry the oily areas, but eventually your sebaceous glands will overcompensate and you'll end up with more oil than you started with. Mild cleansing is best. • Try placing a warm, regular (not decaf) tea bag on a pimple: tea contains tannic acid, which helps to heal breakouts. • Don't squeeze pimples. It's tempting but often makes the problem worse, and it can scar your face. • Fatty foods and chocolate haven't been proven to cause breakouts. Alcohol, tobacco, caffeine, spicy dishes, and iodides are more often the culprits. • One prevention tip: dermatologists say that some cases of chin and cheek acne can be traced to talking on the phone. Clean your receiver at the beginning of the day with alcohol, and try not to rest the phone on your skin.

Sensitive skin. Though skin that's clinically recognized as "sensitive" is fairly rare, many people experience irritation from certain cosmetic ingredients and environmental factors. Keep all the boxes from your cosmetics for a while. If you suspect that a particular product is making you break out, you can show the list of ingredients to a dermatologist to try to isolate the perpetrator. • Sweating can make your skin more prone to irritation; keep this in mind during the summer months and after workouts. • Be sure to remove makeup before working out. Breakouts and similar problems are more common when cosmetics combine with sweat. • Steam baths after a workout can also cause skin irritation. One way to have the best of both worlds is to wear a calming mask in the sauna. • If your skin is very sensitive, steer clear of AHAs and abrasive manual exfoliants. • Often, but not always, certain fragrances found in cosmetics are at the root of irritation. Look for products labeled "fragrance free." "Unscented" merely means that a fragrance has been used to cover up the chemicals' natural smell. • Some preservatives, among them Quaternium-15, Bronopol, and butylated hydroxanisole (BHA), can inflame sensitive skin. They're a lot less common now, replaced by the milder parabens (propyl-, methyl-, and butyl-). If you're still experiencing problems, ask your dermatologist about cosmetics that are preservative-free.

Sunburn. Misery is the best deterrent from getting sunburned twice. Here's how to quell a sunburn: start with any cooling lotion or cool compresses. Use a moisturizing lotion to minimize burning and skin tightness. While researchers aren't unanimously convinced of aloe vera's effectiveness, this product seems to soothe inflammation, inhibit swelling, and allow blood to reach the injured tissue. When looking for cooling lotions, choose one that contains 70 percent aloe vera. You may be tempted to use makeup to cover up redness, but as a general rule, it's better to steer clear of makeup if you have a sunburn. Your skin is more easily irritated and needs time to heal. Sunburn, depending on the degree, usually takes two to five days to clear. Let your dermatologist know about your sunburn history. It may come back as a melanoma decades later.

Wrinkles. Alpha-hydroxy acids (AHAs), the latest weapon in the wrinkle wars, are also effective against age spots and sun damage. Derived from fruits, plants, and sour milk, AHAs are exfoliants: they work by attaching themselves to the dry, dead skin cells on the skin's surface, causing them to flake off. The advantages: AHAs are useful for pregnant women, who shouldn't use Retin-A, which is a vitamin-A derivative that can cause birth defects when taken in high concentrations. And AHAs do not cause the lightening, darkening, or mottling of skin that women with darker complexions have reported with vitamin-A derivatives. The disadvantage: Are AHAs

drugs or cosmetics? So far, AHAs may legally be sold in mild solutions over the counter, as long as companies don't claim on their packaging anything more than glowing, "revived" complexions, but the FDA recently published a report questioning whether AHAs sold over the counter are effective at all. AHA potions in cosmetics range from 1.2 to 5 percent concentrations, but in treatments given by dermatologists, the acid content may go as high as 70 percent. Though generally considered less irritating than Renova and Retin-A, AHAs can still cause reddening and burning, and aren't recommended for sensitive skin.

EYES

Eyebrows. Overplucked eyebrows take three to six weeks to grow back, but if you've been overplucking for years, some hairs may never return. You can make eyebrows appear fuller by using an eyeshadow that matches your natural hair color. Apply it with a fine, stiff eyeliner brush or eyebrow pencil. Use small strokes around and underneath the existing brow, and blend with a small toothbrush. **Tweezing: 1.** A good time to tweeze is after the shower. Since skin is softer then, tweezing is less painful. **2.** Be careful to pluck your eyebrows in the direction they grow. If you pull against the grain, they can grow back sticking straight out instead of lying smoothly against the skin. **3.** Try to tweeze in daylight so you can see what you're doing and avoid the morning-after shock of seeing what you did the night before. **4.** After you tweeze two or three hairs from one brow, do the same to the other. This will help to keep your brows symmetrical. **5.** Don't pluck the hairs above the brow. It will distort the natural line. **6.** Avoid tweezing when

the phone is ringing, the dog needs to be walked, or you've just downed five cups of coffee. **7.** If you take a pencil and hold it vertically right beside your nose, the point where the pencil meets the eyebrow is probably where your brow should start. **8.** If you choose to wax your eyebrows, hairs may grow back sporadically and in different directions.

Eye puffiness. Soak cotton balls in a mixture of half ice water, half cold whole milk, and place one over each eye for 15 minutes. The icy temperature plus the fats in the milk have an anti-inflammatory effect.

Eye redness. Eye drops that promise to "get the red out" use naphazoline, a vasoconstrictor that shrinks the blood vessels artificially, temporarily blanching the white of the eye. Drops should be used only occasionally. If you find yourself using them daily, visit your doctor.

Styes. Caused by bacteria trapped in an eyelash follicle, styes are tender cysts that form at the edge of the eye. If you see one coming, hold a warm, damp washcloth to the area several times a day. Throw away any eye makeup that may have come into contact with the stye, and avoid bringing your fingers to your eyes, because styes are contagious. You might want to make an appointment with an ophthalmologist.

MOUTH

Bad breath. The best defenses against bad breath: brush or scrape your tongue as far back as you can; floss; use mouthwash; be careful with tobacco, alcohol, and coffee; and eat fruits like apples, which cause your mouth to step up saliva production. Saliva helps bad breath by breaking down and encouraging you to swallow food particles that may be causing the problem.

Canker sores. Ulcerous sores on the lips may be the result of the herpes simplex virus or a variety of other causes. If they're herpes sores, they go away in anywhere between a few days and a few weeks without treatment. (The antiviral drug acy-

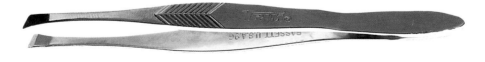

clovir is sometimes prescribed.) But if you find they occur repeatedly, try taking folic acid and B_{12} supplements: sometimes canker sores can result from deficiencies of these two vitamins.

Chapped lips. Lip balm is the best remedy for chapped lips. If you are going to be in the sun, however, use a lip balm with an SPF formula. Lips have no melanin, which means they can't tan, but they can burn—the lower lip is one of the most common sites for skin cancer.

Teeth. It's amazing how much worse a poster model looks after someone's filled in one of her front teeth with a black pen. So brush after every meal, and floss once a day … nag, nag, nag. It's best to avoid over-the-counter hydrogen-peroxide tooth-bleaching products and whitening toothpastes, which can damage—at least temporarily, possibly permanently—the lining of your mouth as well as the very pulp of your teeth. If you must use a whitening agent, calcium peroxide is considered safer than hydrogen peroxide—but if your teeth are stained, it's probably a better idea to talk to your dentist about it first. A couple of dental options: **BONDING** involves the application of a resin over enamel and between teeth to correct irregularities. Think of it as Spackle for the mouth. Bonding lasts three to eight years. **PORCELAIN VENEERING** is like bonding, but more expensive and longer-lasting. The dentist files down the teeth and adheres permanent laminates. Veneering lasts between ten and twenty years.

Cosmetic Surgery

Be glad you weren't considering plastic surgery in the early part of the century, when it was standard procedure to use rubber masks filled with pomade to combat wrinkles, chin straps as a cure for the double chin, and nostril pinchers to reduce the width of your nose. Cosmetic surgery today can be as radical as a full-blown facelift, or as minor as an injection to fill out a frown line or fatten a lip. The trend is toward preventive measures at an earlier age, when the skin is more resilient. Finer tools and advancements in technique have made the big stuff—implants, lifts, and liposuction surgery—less scary as well. As you get older, cosmetic surgery can get more risky. The skin is thinner and may scar more easily. The hairline may be thinner and more receded, making scars more difficult to hide. And medications as benign as aspirin can affect bleeding.

TREATMENT LEXICON

BLEPHAROPLASTY (eyelid surgery): A facelift for the eyelids, in which skin is pulled more tightly, re-draped, and trimmed. Blepharoplasty can erase wrinkles, loose skin, and bags under the eyes; it lasts five to ten years.

BOTOX INJECTIONS: Shots of trace amounts of the botulism toxin into wrinkled areas—between the eyebrows, around the eyes—temporarily paralyzing the muscles underneath and flattening out wrinkles on the forehead.

CELLEX-C: The trademark name for a vitamin C–derived solution that promotes the skin's absorption of vitamin C and fuels the production of collagen; used to reduce the appearance of facial wrinkles and scarring.

CHEMICAL PEELS: These treatments are a serious business. Performed in a doctor's office, they are effective against wrinkling and hyperpigmentation. The problem is, the stronger the peel solution, the greater the skin irritation, and the longer the patient will be out of commission—sometimes over two weeks.

COLLAGEN: A liquid protein that's extracted from cowhide and injected into the inner layers of the skin, filling in fine wrinkles and giving the skin a plumper appearance. The advantage is that the procedure takes no more than 15 minutes and is relatively inexpensive; the disadvantage is that the effects last only about six months, then the process must be repeated. There is also an ongoing controversy in the United States about a possible connection between collagen and autoimmune diseases.

DERMABRASION: Dermabrasion is a serious procedure in which the top layer of skin is removed with a wire brush: it is usually recommended only for deep acne scarring.

DERMAPIGMENTATION: Permanent makeup. Pigments are injected into the dermis in tiny dots, not unlike a tattoo, to approximate a penciled eyelid, lined lip, or sculpted eyebrow.

FACELIFTS: The technology of facelifts is changing rapidly. A few years ago, a facelift was merely a matter of tightening skin over the face and snipping away the excess, which can make a

"I'll go to the bathroom and powder my nose, while you sit here and think of something to say."

UMA THURMAN, *Pulp Fiction*

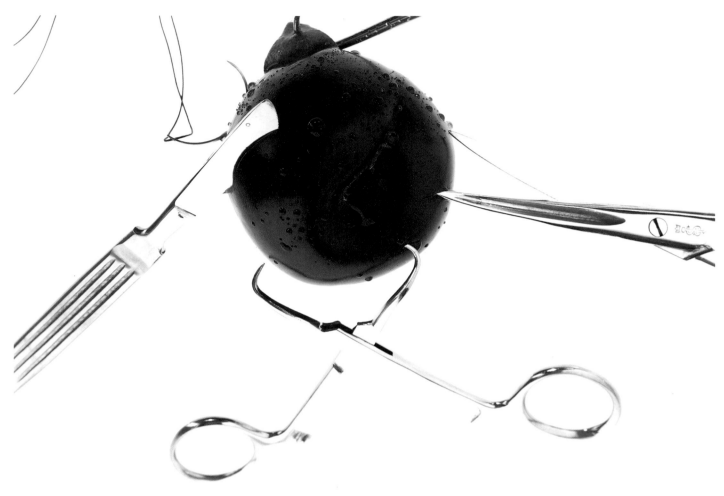

woman look like she's fighting her way through a wind tunnel. These days, fat and muscle underneath the facial skin are being removed and shifted around. The result (sometimes): a face that looks not merely tighter, but … different.

FAT INJECTION: Fat from a patient's own body (usually from the belly) is injected beneath facial wrinkles, in much the same fashion as collagen. There's no risk of an allergic reaction, and not all the fat is remetabolized, so "recharges" aren't so frequent. But it's a more expensive procedure than collagen injections.

LIPOSUCTION: A procedure in which fat is suctioned from the body through a straw called a cannula. Liposuction is the most common form of plastic surgery in the U.S., and is often combined with surgeries like facelifts.

POLYTETRAFLUOROETHYLENE: The same manmade material that your raincoat's made of can plump up your frown lines and the wrinkles that run from your nose to your mouth (officially known as nasolabial folds). Thin threads of Gore-Tex are inserted into the soft tissue just below the skin's surface to prop up the skin.

RETIN-A AND RENOVA: Women have been dabbing themselves with prescription-only Retin-A since 1988; Renova, its milder cousin, is only a few years old. Once used to fight teenage acne, both Retin-A and Renova are powerful exfoliants modeled after vitamin A. They slough off the dead cells that clutter the surface of aging skin and make it look dull. The active ingredient in both is tretinoin, or all-transretinoic acid. They do reverse the fine lines, leathery texture, and age spots caused by the sun, but they also increase the skin's photosensitivity. Renova, which comes in a moisturizing base, can be less irritating than Retin-A. Of course, you have to keep using both indefinitely, or your skin will return to its original appearance. Vitamin-A derivatives such as these should not be used during pregnancy.

"Of course I do all that, darling. That's like going to the dentist. **Why not?** I don't go overboard, but if I can do my eyes, **why not?**"

IRA VON FÜRSTENBERG

where.

By now you're familiar with the "how" of face care and have some ideas on the "what." Now you're ready for the "where." The companies listed here range from large department stores to small boutiques to mail order, so you can shop to suit yourself perfectly.

FREEDOM OF CHOICE

ACADEMY OF FACIAL, PLASTIC, AND RECONSTRUCTIVE SURGERY
800/332-3223
(Advice and referrals for cosmetic surgery)

ALMAY
212/527-4000
(Sun-protection and skin-care products)

AMERICAN BOARD OF DERMATOLOGISTS
313/874-1088
(Skin treatment advice and referrals)

AMERICAN CANCER SOCIETY
212/586-8700
(Information on skin cancer)

ARIZONA NATURAL RESOURCES
602/569-6900
(Antioxidant skin-care line)

AVEDA
800/328-0849
www.aveda.com
(Makeup and skin-care line and salon)

AVON
800/FOR AVON
www.avon.com
(Retail and mail-order makeup and face care)

BANANA REPUBLIC
212/886-7188
(Skin-care products)

BARNEYS NEW YORK
800/777-0087
www.netcity.com/barneysny.html
(Soaps, oils, lotions, perfumes, and sponges)

BATH & BODY WORKS
800/395-1001
(Creams, oils, soaps, lotions)

BENEFIT
800/781-2336
(Makeup and skin-care line)

BIGELOWS
800/793-LIFE
(Wide selection of imported and domestic makeup and skin-care products)

BIOELEMENTS ALPHA-HYDROXY ACID HOTLINE
800/533-3064
(Information on AHAs)

BIOTHERME
888/246-8437
(Body products and facial moisturizers)

BLOOMINGDALE'S
800/777-4999
www.bloomingdales.com
(Skin care, makeup, and boutique)

BOBBI BROWN ESSENTIALS
212/980-7040
www.bobbibrowncosmetics.com
(Makeup and skin-care line)

BODY DRENCH
800/722-2639
(Skin-care and self-tanning products)

THE BODY SHOP
800/541-2535 for orders
www.the-body-shop.com
(Skin-care products with a message)

B2 ACTIGEN
800/784-3633
(Skin-clarifying mask and treatment regimen)

CALVIN KLEIN
800/223-6808
(Skin-care products)

CELLEX-C
800/423-5539
(Prescription-strength antioxidant)

CHAMBERS
800/334-9790
(Vanity mirrors)

CHANEL
908/980-2425
(Skin care)

CHRISTIAN DIOR
212/759-1840
(Makeup line)

CLINIQUE LABS
212/572-3800
www.clinique.com
(Makeup and skin care)

COMPTOIR SUD PACIFIQUE
561/820-9020
(Body and face-care products)

THE COSMETIC FACTORY
800/922-4446
(Makeup line)

ALCONE

Since its birth in 1950 as a supplier of makeup and false eyelashes to showgirls, Alcone has had New York City in its blood. Through its mail-order warehouse, its Manhattan retail outlet, and a little corner of Henri Bendel, Alcone has been instrumental in the explosion of small, high-quality, professional makeup artists' lines: they now stock more than thirty pro lines, to meet the specific needs of makeup artists and customers worldwide. One of our favorites is Cinema Secrets brush cleaner, which cleans and sanitizes brushes instantly, and with a sweet vanilla scent to boot.

(Alcone, 800/466-7446)

KIEHL'S

Kiehl's, a fixture in Manhattan's East Village since 1851, has completely transcended the institution of the modern-day pharmacy. For years they were producers of natural elixirs; later, they were at the forefront of the high-tech manufacture of fluoride and penicillin. In the 1960s, those two worlds met with a new focus on natural skin-care products and cosmetics. Without advertising or fancy packaging—but with expert advice and lots of free samples—Kiehl's has acquired an international following for products like our favorite, Lip Balm No. 1.

(Kiehl's, 800/KIEHLS-1)

COVER GIRL
888/COVER GIRL
www.covergirl.com
(Makeup line)

CRABTREE & EVELYN
800/272-2873
(Skin care, soaps, and lotions)

**DAYTON HUDSON/
MARSHALL FIELD'S**
800/292-2450
(Cosmetics, skin care, and bath products)

DECLEOR USA
800/722-2219
(French aromatherapy and skin care)

DONNA KARAN BEAUTY
800/647-7474
www.donnakaran.com
(Makeup, skin care, and body products)

ECCO BELLA
800/322-9344
(Cruelty-free moisturizing creams, facial cleansers, toners, oils, and perfumes)

ELIZABETH ARDEN
212/261-1000
www.utee.com/arden
(Makeup and skin-care products)

EMPORIO ARMANI
212/727-3240
(Makeup and skin care)

ERBE SALON
800/432-ERBE
(Hypoallergenic, natural skin-care products)

ERNO LASZLO INSTITUTE
800/442-8417
(Skin care)

ESTEE LAUDER
212/572-4433
(Makeup and skin-care lines)

THE GAP
800/GAP STYLE
(Skin-care products)

GARDEN BOTANIKA
800/877-9603
(Face and body scrubs, lotions, and soaps)

GUERLAIN
800/882-8820
(Fragrance, cosmetics, and skin care)

GUINOT
800/444-6621
(Skin-care system)

HENRI BENDEL
212/247-1100
(Skin-care products and makeup)

H₂O PLUS
800/242-BATH
(Bath and skin-care products)

IL MAKIAGE
800/722-1011
(Makeup)

IMAN
800/366-IMAN
(Makeup and skin care for darker complexions)

I NATURAL
212/965-1002
(Makeup and skin care)

JAPONESQUE
800/955-6662
(Professional makeup and tools)

JCPENNEY
800/222-6161
(Makeup and skin-care products)

KIEHL'S
800/KIEHLS-1
(Unique skin-care products)

LANCÔME
800/LANCÔME
www.lancome usa.com
(Makeup and skin-care products)

LA PRAIRIE
800/821-5718
www.laprairie.com
(Skin-care products)

LAURA MERCIER
888/637-2437
(Makeup)

LITE COSMETICS
www.seniorcosmetics.com
(Makeup and skin care for seniors)

LOOK
800/LOOK- 312
(Complete makeup line)

LOOK GOOD, FEEL BETTER
404/329-5763
(Makeup lessons and application for chemotherapy patients)

LORAC
800/845-0705
(Makeup and skin-care products)

LORD & TAYLOR
212/391-3344
(Makeup, skin care, and perfumes)

L'OREAL
212/984-4070
(Makeup and skin-care products)

**LUMINIQUE AT VIDAL
SASSOON**
800/SASSOON
(Custom makeup blending, specializing in discontinued shades)

MAC
800/387-6707
(Makeup, brushes, and accessories)

**MACY'S/BULLOCK'S/
AEROPOSTALE**
800/45 MACYS
www.macys.com
(Makeup, skin care, and perfumes)

MAKE UP FOR EVER
800/757-5175
(Makeup)

MANIC PANIC
800/95-MANIC
(Makeup line)

**MARIO BADESCU SKINCARE
SALON**
800/BADESCU
(Makeup and skin care)

MARSHALL FIELD'S
800/292-2450
(Makeup, skin care, and perfumes)

MARY KAY
800/454-1170
www.marykay.com
(Makeup line)

MASTEY
800/6-MASTEY
(Skin-care products)

MATRIX ESSENTIALS
800/6-MATRIX
(Makeup and skin care)

MAX FACTOR
800/526-8787
(Makeup and skin-care products)

MAYBELLINE
800/944-0730
(Makeup)

MERLE NORMAN STUDIOS
800/40-MERLE
(Beauty supplies)

NAOMI SIMS BEAUTY CENTER
800/556-SIMS
(Makeup and skin care)

**NATURALLY SOOTHING LIP
PROTECTION BALM**
800/NAT-8755
(Naturally soothing lip protection balm)

NEUTROGENA
310/642-1150
(Skin care)

NEIMAN MARCUS
800/937-9146
(Makeup, skin care, and perfumes)

NIVEA
800/937-9146
(Skin care and hypoallergenic moisturizers)

NORDSTROM
800/285-5800
(Makeup, skin care, and perfumes)

NORMA KAMALI BEAUTY
800/4-KAMALI
(Makeup and skin care)

OCEANIQUE
800/567-6751
*(Skin care, including special oil-controlling
toners)*

ON THE ROCKS
800/795-2405
(Insulated makeup bags)

ORIGINS
800/723-7310
(Makeup and skin care)

ORLANE
800/775-2541
(Makeup and skin care)

OSMOTICS
800/440-1411
(Makeup and skin care)

PHILOSOPHY
888/2NEW AGE
*(Environmentally conscious makeup and
skin care)*

POLO/RALPH LAUREN
800/653-7656
(Skin care)

PONDS INSTITUTE
800/34-PONDS
(Face creams)

PRESCRIPTIVES
212/572-4400, x4811
(Makeup, skin care, and color matching)

PRESTIGE
800/722-7488
(Makeup)

**PRINCESS MARCELLA
BORGHESE**
212/572-3100
(Makeup and skin care)

PYCNOGENOL
602/569-6900
(Prescription antioxidant)

REDKEN
212/249-0633
(Makeup and skin care)

REMO (AUSTRALIA)
011/612/331-5007
inforemo@remo.com.au
(Beauty and skin-care products)

REPECHAGE
www.repechage.com
(Seaweed-based skin-care products)

REVLON
800/473-8566
www.revlon.com
(Makeup and skin care)

ST. IVES
800/333-6666
www.stives.com
(Skin care)

SAKS FIFTH AVENUE
212/753-2038
(Makeup and skin care)

SALLY BEAUTY SUPPLY
800/284-SALLY
(Makeup, skin care, and tools)

SENNA
800/537-3662
(Makeup and skin care)

SHISEIDO
800/423-5539
www.shiseido.cojp/index5.htm
(Skin care)

**SHU UEMURA BOUTIQUES
WORLDWIDE**
800/743-8205
(Natural skin care and cosmetics)

SKIN CANCER FOUNDATION
212/725-5176
(Information on sun protection and skin cancer)

SPA THIRA
888/76-THIRA
(Nationwide luxury day spas)

STELLA SALON
888/200-7482
(Soaps and skin-care products)

STILA
800/883-0400
(Makeup-artists' line)

STUDIO GEAR
888/350-GEAR
(Makeup)

TAKASHIMAYA
800/753-2038
(Makeup and skin care)

TARGET STORES
800/800-8800
(Makeup and skin care)

TOM'S OF MAINE
800/985-3874
(Personal-care items)

TRISH McEVOY
800/431-4306
(Makeup and skin care)

TRUCCO
800/829-7322
(Makeup salons)

**OFICINA FARMACEUTICA
DI SANTA MARIA
NOVELLA**

Twelfth-century Dominican
friars may have spent twenty
hours a day in prayer, but
that doesn't mean they didn't
care about their skin.
Florence's Oficina
Farmaceutica, one of the old-
est pharmacies in the world,
can trace its roots directly to
those friars and their extensive knowledge of the healing properties of plants. Not
too many businesses can
claim eight hundred years of
product development. Every
item is handmade and hand-
packaged, and contains only
natural ingredients, like mor-
tar-and-pestle crushed
almonds (for skin softness),
bee pollen (to fight wrinkles), and iris (for oily skin).
Farmaceutica's
products are available in the
U.S. so you don't have to
make a pilgrimage to
get them.

(Takashimaya, 800/753-2038)

TWEEZERMAN
800/645-3340
(Tweezers)

URBAN DECAY COSMETICS
www.urbandecay.com
(Alternative makeup)

VALERIE
800/282-5374
(Lip, brow, and eye-makeup kits)

WALNUT ACRES
800/433-3998
(Organic soaps and moisturizing creams)

YVES SAINT LAURENT
212/246-9494
(Makeup and full skin-care line)

ZHEN COSMETICS
800/457-8455
www.dgi.net/zhen
(Makeup and skin care for Asian women)

NATIONAL LISTINGS

ALABAMA

**DEBORAH STONE SPA
& PARFUMERIE**
3439 Colonnade Parkway
Birmingham, AL 35243
205/957-1177
(Luxury day spa)

INTERLUDES
2415 Canterbury Road
Mt. Brook, AL 35223
205/870-3376
(Specialty makeup and skin care)

PARISIAN
2100 River Chase Galleria
Birmingham, AL 35244
205/987-4200
(Cosmetics, skin-care and bath products)

ARIZONA

GLADABOUT DAY SPAS
6393 East Grant Road
Tucson, AZ 85716
520/885-0000
(Day spa)

ARKANSAS

RANDALL BYARS
5919 Kavanaugh Boulevard
Little Rock, AR 72207
501/664-1008
(Fragrances, soaps, lotions, body aromatherapy, and bath salts)

CALIFORNIA

AROMA VERA
5901 Rodeo Drive
Los Angeles, CA 90016
800/669-9514
(Special face blends and essential oils)

BARE ESSENTIALS
2101 Chestnut Street
San Francisco, CA 94123
(Bath and skin-care products for the entire family)

CRISTINA RADU
8300 Melrose Avenue
Los Angeles, CA 90016
213/655-4020
(Facial-treatment salon)

DAVID STARR
9 Claude Lane
San Francisco, CA 94115
415/421-3223
(Makeup-artists' line of cosmetics)

FILLAMENTO
2185 Fillmore Street
San Francisco, CA 94115
415/931-2224
(Natural soaps and skin care)

FRED SEGAL ENVIRONMENT
8118 Melrose Avenue
Los Angeles, CA 90046
213/651-0239
(Skin care and cosmetics)

KATE ELLIOT BEAUTY BASICS
19826 Ventura Boulevard
Woodland Hills, CA 91364
818/883-4445
(Aromatherapy, soaps, gels, and oils)

LESLIE NORRIS ESTHETIQUE
9009 Beverly Boulevard
West Hollywood, CA 92922
310/888-8820
(Personal facial massage and moisturizing)

LEYDET AROMATICS
Box 2354
Fair Oaks, CA 95628
916/965-7546
("Goddess" blends designed for bath, body, spa, and diffuser)

OAK BALLEY HERB FARM
14648 Pear Tree Lane
Nevada City, CA 95959
916/265-9553
(Herbal extracts, aromatherapy facial kits, and essential oils)

OCEANS OF LOTIONS
842 Cole Street
San Francisco, CA 94117
415/566-2326
(Imported and domestic natural cosmetics)

PALMETTO
1034 Montana Avenue
Santa Monica, CA 90403
310/395-6687
(Natural beauty products)

REAL GOODS TRADING CO.
966 Mazzoni Street
Ukiah, CA 95482
800/762-7325
(Environmental skin-care products)

SCHWARZKOPF
5701 Buckingham Parkway
Culver City, CA 90230
800/234-4672
(Beauty and hair products)

SENNA COSMETICS
367 North Camden Drive
Beverly Hills, CA 90210
310/274-1028
(Makeup artist Eugenia Weston's line of cosmetics)

SIMPLERS BOTANICAL
Box 39
Forestville, CA 95436
707/887-2012
(Herbal preparations, aromatic mists, and essential oils and creams)

SKIN ZONE
575 Castro Street
San Francisco, CA 94114
415/626-7933
(Scented bath oils, colognes, and skin-care products)

STEVEN MILLER
8730 Sunset Boulevard, Suite 200
Los Angeles, CA 90023
310/659-9388
(Facial treatments, specializing in "pore shrinking")

VALERIE SALON
350 North Cañon Drive
Beverly Hills, CA 90210
310/274-7348
(Makeovers)

STILA

Founded by celebrity makeup artist Jeanine Lobell, Stila is about enhancing and concealing features with fewer products and a greater understanding of matching skin tone to Stila's versatile color palette. All of Stila's makeup artists are trained by Lobell herself, and its products were among the first in the industry to be eco-friendly: they're packaged in recycled paper and aluminum, eye pencils are made from 100% recycled paper, and the Stila book, compact, and personalized box are all conveniently refillable. That's because Stila will likely keep you coming back for more.

(Stila, 800/883-0400)

COLORADO

ALFALFA'S MARKET
1645 Broadway
Boulder, CO 80302
303/442-0909
(Fresh and dried botanicals, and all-natural skin-care products)

VELVET SLIPPER
1901 Broadway
Boulder, CO 80302
303/447-1733
(Specialty makeup and skin care)

NEUTROGENA

Eleven minutes after washing with Neutrogena soap, skin returns to its normal pH balance—only one minute longer than washing with water alone. The company was among the first to emphasize medical product research in skin care, designing its soaps with the assistance of dermatologists. Now, in an age in which soap is becoming a four-letter word, Neutrogena's mild formula continues to thrive, and they've branched out into other skin-care products, among them deep cleansers, moisturizers, and self-tanning sprays.

(Neutrogena, 310/642-1150)

CONNECTICUT

CONNECTICUT RIVER TRADING COMPANY
129 Samson Rock Road
Madison, CT 06443
203/245-2481
(Skin-care products)

PARFUMERIE DOUGLAS
51 Main Street
Westport, CT 06880
203/222-9222
(Cosmetics, body lotions, perfumes, and cosmetics cases)

DISTRICT OF COLUMBIA

EFX
1745 Connecticut Avenue
Washington, D.C. 20009
202/462-1300
(Specialty makeup and cosmetics)

FLORIDA

AUTHENTIQUE
3308 Ponce de León Boulevard
Miami, FL 33134
305/446-5424
(Hair removal and waxing)

COSMYL
4401 Ponce de León Boulevard
Miami, FL 33134
305/442-9305
(Facial treatments, featuring aromatherapy, steaming, and massage)

PEUONIA
6285 Bird Road
Miami, FL 33155
305/662-6197
(Electrolysis)

TERRY JACOBS COSMETICS FOR THE TROPICS
4 Grove Isle Drive
Miami, FL 33133
305/856-4066
(Makeup salon and product line specializing in water-based makeup for hot climates)

GEORGIA

NATURAL BODY DAY SPA
1409 North Highland, Suite C
Atlanta, GA 30306
404/872-1039
(Beauty treatments and hair removal)

RICH'S
Lenox Square Shopping Mall
3393 Peachtree Road
Atlanta, GA 30326
404/231-2611
(Fine bath products, fragrances, and scented lotions)

ILLINOIS

FACE & FACIAL CO.
104 East Oak Street
Chicago, IL 60611
312/266-9506
(Facial treatments featuring natural formulas and steam)

MICHAEL THOMAS HAIR SALON AND DAY SPA
1 East Delaware Place
Chicago, IL 60611
312/944-4442
(Hair removal)

INDIANA

EMMET'S
5601 North Illinois
Indianapolis, IN 46205
317/475-0777
(Specialty makeup and skin care)

MASSACHUSETTS

LE PLI AT THE HERITAGE
28 Arlington Street
Boston, MA 02116
617/426-6999
(Facial treatments accompanied by massage)

MICHIGAN

HANAN
31409 Southfield Road
Birmingham, MI 48025
810/644-0277
(Makeup)

NEW MEXICO

WILD OATS
1090 South St. Francis Drive
Santa Fe, NM 87501
505/983-5333
(Skin care and spa therapy)

NEW YORK

ABOUT BODY & FACE
119 West 57th Street
New York, NY 10019
212/586-3990
(Facial treatments and electrolysis)

AD HOC SOFTWARES
410 West Broadway
New York, NY 10012
212/925-2652
(Makeup containers and accessories)

AERO LTD.
132 Spring Street
New York, NY 10012
212/966-1500
(Fine cosmetic accessories)

ALCONE NYC
235 West 19th Street
New York, NY 10011
212/633-0551
(Professional makeup artists' specialty store)

ANUSKA DAY SPA
241 East 60th Street
New York, NY 10022
212/355-6404
(Skin-care and cellulite clinic)

ARISTA SURGICAL SUPPLY
67 Lexington Avenue
New York, NY 10010
212/679-3694
(Makeup tools)

AVEDA SALON & SPA
456 West Broadway
New York, NY 10012
212/473-0280
(Professional facials, skin care, and makeup products)

BATH ISLAND
469 Amsterdam Avenue
New York, NY 10024
212/787-9415
(Bath, body, skin, and hair-care products)

BLISS SPA
569 Broadway
New York, NY 10012
212/219-8970
(Facial treatments and skin care to suit)

BUMBLE & BUMBLE
146 East 56th Street
New York, NY 10022
212/521-6500
(Professional makeup artists)

CARAPAN
5 West 16th Street
New York, NY 10011
212/633-6220
(Professional facials)

CASWELL-MASSEY
518 Lexington Avenue
New York, NY 10017
212/755-2254
(Skin care, makeup, and soaps)

CITIZEN HEALTH & BEAUTY AIDS
541 Broadway
New York, NY 10012
212/219-3467
(Discounted makeup and skin care)

DEAN & DELUCA
560 Broadway
New York, NY 10012
212/431-1691
(Fresh herbs and fruits ideal for homemade skin care)

ELECTROLYSIS BY MARIA
990 Avenue of the Americas
New York, NY 10018
212/947-1542
(Electrolysis)

ELIZABETH ARDEN RED DOOR SALON
691 Fifth Avenue
New York, NY 10020
212/546-0200
(Professional facials)

ERBE
196 Prince Street
New York, NY 10012
212/966-1445
(Herbal beauty center)

EVOLUTION
120 Spring Street
New York, NY 10012
212/343-1114
(Cosmetic accessories)

FACE STOCKHOLM
110 Prince Street
New York, NY 10012
212/334-3900
(Makeup and skin care)

FELISSIMO
10 West 56th Street
New York, NY 10019
212/956-4438
(Soaps, gels, and lotions)

FREDERIC FEKKAI BEAUTE DE PROVENCE
15 East 57th Street
New York, NY 10022
212/753-9500
(Complete beauty treatments)

GEORGETTE KLINGER SKIN CARE SALONS
501 Madison Avenue
New York, NY 10022
212/838-3200
(Full skin-treatment salon)

GOODEBODIES
330 Columbus Avenue
New York, NY 10023
212/721-9317
(Bath oils and gels)

GREENLIFE
400 West Broadway
New York, NY 10012
(Natural, environmentally friendly lotions, shampoos, and skin-care products)

GURNEY'S INN
Old Montauk Highway
Montauk, NY
516/668-2345
(Luxury day spa)

IL MAKIAGE
107 East 60th Street
New York, NY 10022
212/371-3992
(Salon, in-house makeup, and skin-care lines)

ILONA OF HUNGARY
629 Park Avenue
New York, NY 10021
212/288-5155
(Skin-care institute specializing in facials and massage)

JANET SARTIN INSTITUTE OF SKIN CARE
500 Park Avenue
New York, NY 10022
212/794-2961
(Facial treatments)

KOZUÉ AESTHETIC SPA
795 Madison Avenue
New York, NY 10021
212/734-8600
(Professional facials)

LING SKIN CARE
128 Thompson Street
New York, NY 10012
212/982-8833
(Herbal facials accompanied by massage)

MARIO BADESCU SKIN CARE
320 East 52nd Street
New York, NY 10022
212/758-1065
(Makeup and skin-care products)

ORIGINS FEEL-GOOD SPA
The Sports Center (Pier 60)
Chelsea Piers
New York, NY 10011
212/336-6780
(Professional facials)

PENINSULA SPA
700 Fifth Avenue, 21st Floor
New York, NY 10020
212/903-3910
(Professional facials)

PHYTOLOGIE
625 Madison Avenue
New York, NY 10022
800/648-0349
(Botanical beauty products)

PORTICO BED & BATH
139 Spring Street
New York, NY 10012
212/579-9500
(Soaps, oils, and scrubs)

REPECHAGE SARKLI LTD.
1037 Third Avenue
New York, NY 10001
212/319-1770
(Facials, specializing in seaweed treatment)

RICKY'S
590 Broadway
New York, NY 10012
212/226-5552
(Discounted makeup and skin care)

SALON ISHI
70 East 55th Street
New York, NY 10022
212/888-ISHI
(Skin care and shiatsu massage)

SKIN CARE CLINIC
162 West 56th Street, Suite 206
New York, NY 10019
212/582-5720
(Hair removal and herbal wax)

SCREENFACE

The two Screenface makeup studios, both located in London's hip Notting Hill district, are cosmetic fun houses, filled with one of the most diverse and extensive product lines in the world. Screenface is the leading cosmetic supplier to the British film industry: along with flight-proof makeup boxes, famous PVC-vinyl zip cases, handmade brushes, and innovative sponges, you can buy cans of phony blood, beards, and temporary tattoos. Screenface cosmetics come in a wide range of shades and textures that have been formulated to cover the rigors of a film shoot and the rigors of your day. The studios are staffed by professional makeup artists who can provide purchasing and application tips and full makeovers.

(Screenface, 011/44/171/221-8289)

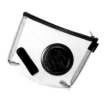

LE CLERC

Paris-based Le Clerc produces the most famous face powder in the world—actually, twenty-five different shades of it, to match every skin tone to a tee. Its consistency is superfine because of its relatively low talc content. Instead it's formulated with rice flour, which is softer and finer, and creates remarkably sheer, transparent coverage. Banane, a yellow-toned powder, is Le Clerc's most popular shade, and works best on fair to medium skins. For years Le Clerc products were nearly impossible to find outside of France and professional makeup artists' kits, but now they can be found at better stores worldwide, among them Bigelows.

(Bigelows, 800/793-LIFE)

SUSAN CIMINELLI DAY SPA
601 Madison Avenue
New York, NY 10022
212/688-5500
(Facial treatments)

TERRA VERDE TRADING CO.
120 Wooster Street
New York, NY 10012
212/925-4533
(Environmentally safe beauty products)

THE VITAMIN SHOPPE
375 Avenue of the Americas
New York, NY 10011
212/929-6553
(Vitamins)

WIN TROPICAL AQUARIUM
169 Mott Street
New York, NY 10013
212/343-2875
(Seaweed)

ZITOMER PHARMACY
969 Madison Avenue
New York, NY 10021
212/737-4480
(Travel-size cosmetics and toiletries)

ZONA
97 Greene Street
New York, NY 10012
212/925-6750
(Skin-care products)

NORTH CAROLINA

POSSIBILITIES
157 South Stratford Road
Winston-Salem, NC 27104
910/721-1022
(Specialty makeup and skin care)

OHIO

A SHADE ABOVE
Beachcliff Market Square
19300 Detroit Road
Rocky River, OH 44116
216/356-0604
(Specialty makeup and skin care)

OREGON

EARTHEN JOYS
1412 Eleventh Street
Astoria, OR 97103
503/325-0426
(Bath and body products)

PENNSYLVANIA

THE SPA AT PAUL & KAY'S
264 South Twentieth Street
Philadelphia, PA 19103
215/732-6176
(Facial treatments, specializing in hydrotherapy)

TENNESSEE

ZOE
4564 Poplar
Memphis, TN 38117
901/821-9900
(Specialty makeup and skin care)

TEXAS

ERICA'S
4803 West Lovers Lane
Dallas, TX 75209
214/352-9406
(High-tech facial treatments)

PATRICIA'S DAY SPA
6000 Broadway
San Antonio, TX 78209
210/829-1969
(Luxury day spa)

THE SPA AT THE FOUR SEASONS
4150 North MacArthur Boulevard
Irving, TX 75038
214/717-2401
(Facial spa at the Four Seasons resort)

UTAH

POTIONS & LOTIONS
381 Trolley Square
Salt Lake City, UT 84102
801/355-1609
(Face-care products)

WASHINGTON

GENE JUAREZ SALON
690 Tacoma Mall
4502 South Steele
Tacoma, WA 98409
206/323-7773
(Day spa)

INTERNATIONAL LISTINGS

AUSTRALIA

GEORGES AUSTRALIA LTD.
162 Collins Street
Melbourne
3/283-5555
(Bath and beauty products)

GRACE BROS.
436 George Street
Sydney
2/218-1111

HARBOURSIDE
Darling Harbour
Sydney
2/552-0261
(Skin-care products and boutique)

CANADA

OGILVY
1307 St. Catherine Street West
Montreal H3G 1P7
514/842-7711
(Soaps, lotions, and cosmetics)

FRANCE

ANNICK GOUTAL
14 rue de Castiglione
Paris 75001
0142/60-52-82
(Skin care and cosmetics)

GALERIES LAFAYETTE
40 boulevard Haussmann
Paris 75009
0142/82-34-56
(Skin care and cosmetics)

L'AROMARINE
45 rue Saint-Louis-en-l'Ile
Paris 75004
0146/34-26-32
(Skin care and cosmetics)

SANTOLINE
34 boulevard Victor-Hugo
13210 St. Rémy de Provence
90/92-11-96
(Skin care and cosmetics)

YVES ROCHER
238 rue de Rivoli
Paris 75001
0142/97-53-29
(Natural skin care and cosmetics)

GERMANY

MEY & EDLICH
Theatinerstrasse 7
Munich
89/290-0590
(Bath and skin-care products)

SELBACH
Kürfürstendamm 159
Berlin
30/883-2526
(Makeup and skin-care products)

GREAT BRITAIN

THE BODY SHOP INTERNATIONAL
Watersmead, Littlehampton,
West Sussex, BN17 6LS
190/373-1500
(Bath and skin-care products)

COSMETICS TO GO
Freepost, Poole, Dorset
BH15 1BR
120/262-1966
(Bath and skin-care products)

CRABTREE & EVELYN, LTD.
55–57 South Edwardes Square
London W8 6HP
171/603-1611
(Body, bath, and face-care products)

HARRODS
87–135 Brompton Road
Knightsbridge
London SW1X 7XL
171/730-1234
(Skin-care products)

HARVEY NICHOLS
109–125 Knightsbridge
London SW1X 7RJ
171/235 5000
(Makeup and skin-care products)

HEALS
196 Tottenham Court Road
London W1A1 BJ
171/235-5000
(Bath and skin-care products)

HOUSE OF FRASER
171/834-1515 for U.K. stores
(Bath and skin-care products)

JOHN LEWIS
278 Oxford Street
London W1A 1EX
171/629-7711
(Bath and skin-care products)

LIBERTY
210–220 Regent Street
London W1R 6AH
171/734-1234
(Makeup and skin-care products)

MARKS & SPENCER
99 Kensington High Street
London W8 5SQ
171/938-3711
(Bath and skin-care products)

MUJI
29 Great Marlborough Street
London W1V 1HL

171/494-1197
(No–name brand bath and skin-care products and containers)

NEAL'S YARD REMEDIES
5 Golden Cross
Cornmarket Street
Oxford OX1 3EU
186/524-5436
(Natural beauty products and supplies)

PENHALIGON'S
16 Burlington Arcade
Piccadilly
London W1
171/629-1416
(Bath and skin-care products)

SCREENFACE
20 & 24 Powis Terrace
Westbourne Park Road
London W11 1JH
171/221-8289
(Professional makeup artists' specialty store)

SELFRIDGES
400 Oxford Street
London W1A 1AB
171/629-1234
(Bath and skin-care products)

SPACE NK
41 Earlham Street
Thomas Neals
Covent Garden
London WC2H 9LD
171/379-7030
(Makeup and skin-care products, specializing in American cosmetic lines)

ITALY

OFICINA FARMACEUTICA DE LA PIAZZA SANTA MARIA NOVELLA
via della Scala, 16
Florence
55/230-2437
(Natural and custom-blended cosmetics and skin-care products)

JAPAN

ISETAN
3-14-1 Shinjuku-ku
Shinjuku-ku 160 Tokyo
3/3352-1111
(Makeup and skin-care products)

MITSUKOSHI
1-4-1 Nihombashi
Muromachi
Chuo ku, 103 01 Tokyo
3/3241-3311
(Makeup and skin-care products)

MUJIRUSHI
5-50-6 Jingumae
Shibuya-ku, 150 Tokyo
3/3407-4666
(No–name brand cosmetics and skin-care products)

PARCO
15-1 Udagawa-cho
Shibuya-ku, 150 Tokyo
3/3464-5111
(Makeup and skin-care products)

TAKASHIMAYA
2-4-1 Nihombashi
Chuo-ku, 103 Tokyo
3/3211-4111
(Makeup and skin-care products)

TINAMARRY
20-13 Sarugakucho
Shibuya-ku, 150 Tokyo
3/5789-9800
(Makeup and skin-care products)

MAKEUP AND SKIN CARE ON THE INTERNET

PAULA BEGOUN ("THE COSMETICS COP")
www.cosmeticscop.com
(Reviews and advice on makeup and skin-care products)

COSMETICS CONNECTION
www.kleinman.com/cosmetic/index.html
(Makeup and skin-care related reviews, advice, and links)

A FASHION EXPERIENCE: COSMETICS AND SKIN CARE
www.cosmetics.com
(Information, product reviews, and ordering site)

THE LIPSTICK PAGE
www.users.wineasy.sc/bjornt/lip.html
(Review of lipsticks)

MAKEUP SWAP
www.internetisland.com/swap/
("Trade what you don't want for what you do with fellow makeup junkies.")

ONLINE BEAUTY SHOP
http://members.hknet.com/~utc/utc.htm
(Makeup and skin-care product ordering site)

ONLINE COSMETICS
www.fia.net/la/cg/cosmetics/skincare/
(Cosmetic tips, reviews, and product ordering)

SALON KENNICE BASHAR
www.hair-beauty-products.com/
(Makeup and skin-care ordering site)

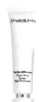

ELIZABETH ARDEN

One of the most popular
and versatile beauty products in history, Elizabeth
Arden's Eight Hour Creme
has been soothing dry skin,
sunburns, scrapes, tough
cuticles, and chapped
lips for the better part
of this century.

In 1916, Arden's then-
fledgling company was the
first in America to create a
complete line of makeup
and skin-care products.
The Eight Hour Creme fit
all skin types and quickly
became the line's corner-
stone and a symbol of
Elizabeth Arden's innova-
tive harmony of tradition
and technology. Its miracle-
working reputation was
solidified once and for all
in 1947, when Miss Arden's
horse, Jet Pilot, won the
Kentucky Derby.
Her trainer's secret?
Regular hoof treatments
with Eight Hour Creme.

(Elizabeth Arden, 212/261-1000)

Resources

Quotes

2 Cynthia Heimel, *Sex Tips for Girls* (Fireside Books, 1983).

14 F. Scott Fitzgerald, "Bernice Bobs Her Hair" (1920), from *The Stories of F. Scott Fitzgerald* (Collier, 1986).

16 Anna Magnani, as quoted in *An Encyclopedia of Women's Wit, Anecdotes and Stories*, edited by Cathy Handley (Prentice Hall, 1982).

22 Groucho Marx, as quoted in *Bartlett's Familiar Quotations* (Little, Brown, 1992).

26 Ernest Hemingway, *A Moveable Feast* (Scribner's, 1964).

34 Abraham Lincoln, as quoted in *The 21st Century Dictionary of Quotations*, edited by the Princeton Language Institute (Philip Lief Group, 1993).

46 Andy Warhol, *The Philosophy of Andy Warhol: From A to B and Back Again* (Harcourt Brace, 1975).

50 Stéphane Marais, as quoted in "Monsieur Makeup," by Heidi Lender, *W*, May 1994.

59 Tracy Young, *Allure*, August 1995.

63 Woody Allen, as quoted in *This Is Really a Great City (I Don't Care What Anybody Says)*, by J. P. Fennell (Citadel Press, 1991).

64 Courtney Love, "Doll Parts," on Hole, *Live Through This* (DGC, 1994).

70 Claudia Shear, *Blown Sideways Through Life* (Dial Press, 1995).

80 Emma Thompson, as quoted in *People*, September 6, 1993.

82 Budd Schulberg, *What Makes Sammy Run?* (Modern Library, 1941).

90 Calvin Klein, as quoted in *The New York Times*, March 6, 1977.

97 Ring Lardner, as quoted in *The 1,911 Best Things Anybody Ever Said*, edited by Robert Byrne (Fawcett Columbine, 1988).

100 RuPaul, *Lettin' It All Hang Out* (Hyperion, 1995).

105 Andy Warhol, *The Philosophy of Andy Warhol: From A to B and Back Again* (Harcourt Brace, 1975).

114 William Shakespeare, *Macbeth*, as quoted in *Bartlett's Familiar Quotations* (Little, Brown, 1992).

120 George V. Higgins, as quoted in the *Wall Street Journal*, July 8, 1984.

125 F. Scott Fitzgerald, *This Side of Paradise* (Scribner's, 1920).

131 Crystal Gayle, "Don't It Make My Brown Eyes Blue" (Curb Records, 1990).

133 Liz Phair, "Supernova," from *Whip-Smart* (Matador Records, 1994).

139 Jerry Seinfeld, as quoted in *Just Joking*, by Ronald L. Smith and Jon Winokur (WordStar International, 1992).

144 Anaïs Nin, *A Spy in the House of Love* (Pocket Books, 1994).

167 Donna Karan, as quoted in *Harper's Bazaar*, July 1994.

170 Charles Revson, as quoted in *The 21st Century Dictionary of Quotations*, edited by the Princeton Language Institute (Philip Lief Group, 1993).

175 Uma Thurman in *Pulp Fiction*, screenplay by Quentin Tarantino, Miramax Films, 1994.

177 Ira von Fürstenberg, as quoted in "The Real Princess," *W*, December 1995.

192 Coco Chanel, as quoted in *What is Beauty?* (Universe Publishing, 1997).

INDEX

CHIC SIMPLE STAFF

PARTNERS Kim & Jeff
ASSISTANT EDITOR Will Georgantas
PRODUCTION ASSOCIATE Jinger Peissig
OFFICE MANAGER Gillian Oppenheim
COPY EDITOR Borden Elniff
PRESIDENT, CHIC SIMPLE INTERNATIONAL Steve Diener

ACKNOWLEDGMENTS

SPECIAL THANKS TO: Claire Bradley Ong, Gabrielle Brooks, Amy Capen, Dori Carlson, Robin Cavan, Alicia Cheng, Althea Cox, Franc Cussoneau, Anna DeLuca, Damian Donck, Richela Fabian, Beau Friedlander, Jane Friedman, Stefan Friedman, Hedy Gold, Robin Grimes, Kate Doyle Hooper, Andy Hughes, Carol Janeway, Pat Johnson, Regina Kulic, Nicholas Latimer, Morise Cabasso and Elena Arboleda at Mario Badescu, Sonny Mehta, Celeste Lambert, Babs Lefrak, Bill Loverd, Brenda Lynn, Christine Notaro, Philip Patrick, Carla Phillips, Marcy Posner, Mona Reilly, Tracy Rose, Amy Schuler, Mel Semensky, Diane Shaw, Kathy Shore-Sirotin, Suzanne Smith, Takuyo Takahashi, Shelley Wanger, Helen Watt, Katherine Wessling, Amy Zenn. HAIR STYLING throughout book by Isabel Lazo, Matteo Manetti, and Sabrina Meyers at Bumble and Bumble, New York City.

INVALUABLE RESOURCES

Some of the best resources for the most up-to-date advances in makeup and skin care are magazines. We found the following resources especially enlightening: *Allure*; *Cosmopolitan*; Kate de Castelbajac, *The Face of the Country: 100 Years of Makeup and Style* (Rizzoli, 1995); Dr. Hauschka Cosmetics; *Seasons* newsletter; *Harper's Bazaar*; Rex Hilverdink and Diana Lewis Jewell, *Making Up* (Clarkson Potter, 1986); Carole Jackson, *Color Me Beautiful Makeup Book* (Ballantine, 1987); Dr. Barney Kenet and Patricia Lawler, *Saving Your Skin* (Turnaround, 1994); *Mademoiselle*; *Marie Claire*; Mario Badescu Skincare; *Mirabella*; *The New York Times Magazine*; Nelson Lee Novick, M.D., *You Can Look Younger at Any Age* (Henry Holt & Co., 1996); *Self*; *Vogue*; *W*.

COMMUNICATIONS

Chic Simple is about information, and you, dear reader, are an essential conduit to that information. Since the publication of our first books, the letters, E-mail, and faxes have pointed out everything from typos to unique stores and products from all over the globe. With your feedback have come suggestions that have resulted in entire Chic Simple titles-by-request. So please write to us at:

CHIC SIMPLE
84 WOOSTER STREET
NEW YORK, NY 10012
Fax: (212) 343-9678
E-mail: info@chicsimple.com
AOL address: ChicSimple
Website: http://www.chicsimple.com
Stay in touch because . . .
"The more you know,
the less you need."

Please share with us any skin-care or makeup secrets that make your life easier.

A NOTE ON THE TYPE

The text of this book was set in New Baskerville and Futura. The ITC version of **NEW BASKERVILLE** is called Baskerville, which itself is a facsimile reproduction of types cast from molds made by John Baskerville (1706–75) from his designs. Baskerville's original face was one of the forerunners of the type style known to printers as "modern face"—a "modern" of the period 1800. **FUTURA** was produced in 1928 by Paul Renner (1878–1956), former director of the Munich School of Design, for the Bauer Type Foundry. Futura is simple in design and wonderfully restful to the eye. It has been widely used in advertising because of its even, modern appearance in mass and its harmony with a great variety of other modern types. Additional display faces: **INTERSTATE** is based on the signage alphabets of the U.S. Federal Highway Administration. Tobias Frere-Jones designed Interstate in 1993, and in 1994 expanded it for The Font Bureau, Inc., a typographic foundry in Boston, Massachusetts. **HTF LEVIATHAN** by The Hoefler Type Foundry, Inc. of New York City is a modern font based on nineteenth-century type styles.

SEPARATIONS AND
FILM PREPARATION BY
PROFESSIONAL GRAPHICS
Rockford, Illinois

PRINTED AND BOUND BY
BUTLER & TANNER, LTD.
Frome, England

HARDWARE

Power PC 9500, 8100, Apple Macintosh Power PC 8100, Quadra 800 personal computers; APS Technologies Syquest Drives; Iomega Zip Drive; MicroNet DAT drive; SuperMac 21-inch color monitor; Radius PrecisionColor Display/20; Radius 24X series video board; QMS 1660 printer; Hewlett-Packard LaserJet 4; Global Village OneWorld modem; Braun FlavorSelect KF 145B.

SOFTWARE

QuarkXPress 3.3, Adobe Photoshop 2.5.1, Microsoft Word 5.1, FileMaker Pro 2.0, Adobe Illustrator 5.0.1.

MUSICWARE

The Beach Boys (*Pet Sounds*), Buckwheat Zydeco (*On a Night Like This*), The Cardigans (*First Band on the Moon*), The Clash (*London Calling*), John Coltrane (*Newport '63*), *Cowabunga! The Surf Box*, Dead Can Dance (*Spiritchaser*), The Flatlanders (*More a Legend than a Band*), The Grateful Dead (*You Name It*), The Harder They Come (*Motion Picture Soundtrack*), Jutta Hipp with Zoot Sims, Chris Isaak (*San Francisco Days*), Moby (*Everything Is Wrong*), Tom Petty and the Heartbreakers (*Greatest Hits*), Liz Phair (*Exile in Guyville*), The Rolling Stones (*Beggar's Banquet, Let It Bleed, Sticky Fingers, Exile on Main Street*), Sonny Rollins (*Saxophone Colossus*), Roxy Music (*Siren*), Saint Etienne (*So Tough*), Son Volt (*Trace*), Bruce Springsteen (*The Wild, the Innocent, and the E Street Shuffle*), Tobin Sprout (*Carnival Boy*), The Sugarcubes (*Life's Too Good*), Bunny Wailer (*Blackheart Man*), Dinah Washington (*The Complete Dinah Washington on Mercury*), The Youngbloods (*Elephant Mountain*).

CLOTHES

BODY

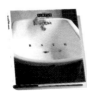

HOME

COOKING

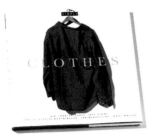

WOMEN'S WARDROBE

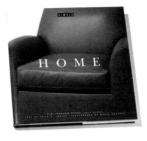

WORK CLOTHES

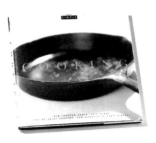

BED LINENS

EYEGLASSES

SCARVES

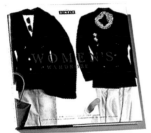

ACCESSORIES

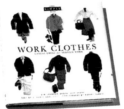

PACKING

COOKING TOOLS

DESK

SHIRT AND TIE

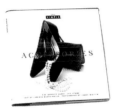
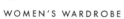

SCENTS

TOOLS

BATH

PAINT

NURSERY

STORAGE